Patients' Guide to
Lymphoma

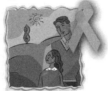

Aditya Bardia, MD, MPH

Clinical Fellow
Department of Medical Oncology
The Sidney Kimmel Comprehensive Cancer Center
Johns Hopkins University School of Medicine
Baltimore, MD

Eric J. Seifter, MD, FACP

Associate Professor of Medicine and Oncology
The Sidney Kimmel Comprehensive Cancer Center
Johns Hopkins University School of Medicine
Baltimore, MD

SERIES EDITORS
Lillie D. Shockney, RN, BS, MAS

University Distinguished Service Associate Professor of Breast Cancer;
Administrative Director of Breast Cancer; Associate Professor, Department of Surgery; Associate
Professor, Department of Obstetrics and Gynecology, Johns Hopkins School of Medicine; Associate
Professor, Johns Hopkins School of Nursing
Baltimore, MD

Gary R. Shapiro, MD

Chairman, Department of Oncology
Johns Hopkins Bayview Medical Center
Director, Johns Hopkins Geriatric Oncology Program
The Sidney Kimmel Comprehensive Cancer Center at Johns Hopkins
Baltimore, MD

JONES AND BARTLETT PUBLISHERS
Sudbury, Massachusetts
BOSTON   TORONTO   LONDON   SINGAPORE

World Headquarters

Jones and Bartlett Publishers
40 Tall Pine Drive
Sudbury, MA 01776
978-443-5000
info@jbpub.com
www.jbpub.com

Jones and Bartlett Publishers
Canada
6339 Ormindale Way
Mississauga, Ontario L5V 1J2
Canada

Jones and Bartlett Publishers
International
Barb House, Barb Mews
London W6 7PA
United Kingdom

Jones and Bartlett's books and products are available through most bookstores and online booksellers. To contact Jones and Bartlett Publishers directly, call 800-832-0034, fax 978-443-8000, or visit our website, www.jbpub.com.

Substantial discounts on bulk quantities of Jones and Bartlett's publications are available to corporations, professional associations, and other qualified organizations. For details and specific discount information, contact the special sales department at Jones and Bartlett via the above contact information or send an email to specialsales@jbpub.com.

The authors, editor, and publisher have made every effort to provide accurate information. However, they are not responsible for errors, omissions, or for any outcomes related to the use of the contents of this book and take no responsibility for the use of the products and procedures described. Treatments and side effects described in this book may not be applicable to all people; likewise, some people may require a dose or experience a side effect that is not described herein. Drugs and medical devices are discussed that may have limited availability controlled by the Food and Drug Administration (FDA) for use only in a research study or clinical trial. Research, clinical practice, and government regulations often change the accepted standard in this field. When consideration is being given to use of any drug in the clinical setting, the healthcare provider or reader is responsible for determining FDA status of the drug, reading the package insert, and reviewing prescribing information for the most up-to-date recommendations on dose, precautions, and contraindications, and determining the appropriate usage for the product. This is especially important in the case of drugs that are new or seldom used.

Production Credits
Executive Publisher: Christopher Davis
Editorial Assistant: Sara Cameron
Production Director: Amy Rose
Production Assistant: Tina Chen
Senior Marketing Manager: Barb Bartoszek
V.P., Manufacturing and Inventory Control: Therese Connell
Cover Design: Kristin E. Parker
Cover Image: © ImageZoo/age fotostock
Composition: Appingo Publishing Services
Printing and Binding: Malloy, Inc.
Cover Printing: Malloy, Inc.

Library of Congress Cataloging-in-Publication Data
Bardia, Aditya.
Johns Hopkins patients' guide to lymphoma / Aditya Bardia, Eric J. Seifter; series editors, Lillie D. Shockney, Gary R. Shapiro.
   p. cm.—(Johns Hopkins patients' guide)
Includes index.
ISBN 978-0-7637-8513-0
1. Lymphomas—Diagnosis. 2. Lymphomas—Treatment. I. Seifter, Eric J. II. Title.
RC280.L9B36 2010
616.99'462—dc22

                                                            2009042296

6048

Printed in the United States of America
14 13 12 11 10   10 9 8 7 6 5 4 3 2 1

CONTENTS

PREFACE

I t is astounding to consider how dismal the prognosis was for patients with Hodgkin's or non-Hodgkin's lymphomas a mere 60 years ago. During the 1960s and 70s, physicians were amazed by successes achieved with combinations of chemotherapy agents and radiotherapy. The majority of patients diagnosed today, even in advanced stages, can expect either to be cured or to live good quality lives for many productive years.

A diagnosis of any malignancy is overwhelming, and is no less so for those with lymphoma; however, most individuals will have excellent responses to modern therapies, while research continues to uncover breakthroughs every year.

This book is meant as a guide and supplement for you and your family. Empowering yourself with knowledge can help inform your decisions about treatment choices. Most of all, you should gain confidence about the available therapies and your own prognosis. This book is part of the *Johns Hopkins Patients' Guide* series designed to educate patients about their cancer diagnosis and the treatments that will be proposed. We hope this information will guide you and your support teams of family, friends, and providers.

Aditya Bardia, MD, MPH

Eric J. Seifter, MD, FACP

DEDICATION

This book is dedicated to all our lymphoma patients and their families and friends. Your courage and determination amaze us every day.

I would like to thank my wife, Vibha, and my son, Omav, for their help, patience, and constant encouragement.

—AB

I would like to thank my team of "angels" who care so well for my patients and who reviewed many sections of this book and provided valuable comments:

Dawn Guttman, Jackie Neun, Anna Recchio, and Lauren Wirth.

—EJS

Introduction

How to Use This Book for Your Benefit

The goal of this book is to help you learn more about your cancer and make informed decisions about your care. By being better informed, we hope that you will be able to better confront the challenges ahead as you proceed through treatment and recovery. You will receive a lot of information from your healthcare team and will probably seek out some information on the Internet or in bookstores. No doubt friends and family members, meaning well, will attempt to give you advice about what to do and when to do it, and try to steer you in certain directions. Relax. Yes, your doctor has told you that you have lymphoma. Although the diagnosis of lymphoma is frightening, there is hope. There are more people surviving lymphoma today than ever before. Hearing the diagnosis is difficult, but by empowering yourself with support and accurate information, you can participate in the decision making about your care and treatment.

This book is designed to be a how-to guide that takes you through the various treatment options and side effects, and will help you put together a plan of action so that you become a lymphoma survivor. The book contains information about current treatment options as well as recommendations for living with and surviving cancer. There is also an index in the back and resources listed for your further review and information. This information will help you to understand the how, when, and why of treatment options so you are in a much better position to be able to make treatment decisions with your doctors. Let's begin now with understanding what has happened and what the first steps are to get you well again.

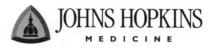

FIRST STEPS—
I'VE BEEN DIAGNOSED
WITH LYMPHOMA

You have recently had a lymph node biopsy or have been told by your primary physician that the lymph nodes on the CAT (computerized axial tomography) scan look like lymphoma. No doubt you are in shock having heard those words. It is natural to think such things as, "I don't have a family history, so how is this possible? I don't have any risk factors, so how did I get it?" So consider these facts: According to the American Cancer Society, one in three people in the United States will develop some type of cancer in their lifetime. Lymphoma is the fifth most common cancer among men and women. Unlike some other tumors, family history does not play an important role in the development of lymphoma. In fact, the risk factors for lymphoma are largely unknown. Trying to guess them will exhaust you. It exhausts the researchers who are working hard to try to discover them on your behalf.

HOW TO SELECT YOUR ONCOLOGY TEAM

You want to be in the hands of experts. This isn't a simple gallbladder problem or hernia repair. This is cancer! Don't rely on self-promoting advertisements on television either as your way to select a facility and doctor. A personal physician, friends, relatives, or neighbors can point you toward the best oncologists and the best cancer centers in your area. Major cancer centers are designated by the National Cancer Institute as part of the NCCN (National Comprehensive Cancer Network), and are good sources for care or for second opinions. However, many community hospitals and community oncologists are affiliated with these regional centers and can provide the same level of expertise and personal care. For management of lymphomas, the team concept is less important than finding the right "quarterback" who shares your values and commitment for getting well. Deciding on the right course of action can be challenging since many different routes may reach the same good result, but with differences in side effects. It is important to have the right person to discuss these options with you.

It's not unusual to get a second opinion after an initial consultation, particularly if the provider or facility does not have expertise in lymphoma management.

While it is not wrong to "shop around" until you find an office or program that meets your needs based on location, expertise, and the compassionate care you sense in the providers, be careful not to get too many opinions as it will likely confuse you and waste crucial time as well. One good tip is that the most experienced providers involved with lymphomas are members of two societies: the American Society of Clinical Oncology (ASCO: http://www.asco.org)

and the American Society of Hematology (ASH: http://www.hematology.org). Both of these societies list their members and the best physicians and nurse practitioners usually belong to these groups. Further resources are listed in Chapter 11.

GATHERING RECORDS: BIOPSY, RADIOLOGY STUDIES, AND OTHER TESTS

As soon as you hear the words, "You have lymphoma," request a copy of your scans and the pathology. These are the two most critical items. Be sure to obtain copies of all your medical records and request copies as you continue this journey so you maintain your own portfolio of treatment and test results. Begin with the initial scans or X-rays that found the worrisome mass or lymph nodes. If you have had a biopsy, gather the pathology reports. Your doctor may also want to see any radiology reports from the last 3 years. No matter who sees you—surgeon, medical oncologist, or radiation oncologist—they will want to review these reports. Although a report of the findings is helpful, it is also beneficial for them to review the actual films or images taken. Find out from the facility where the imaging was done how to go about picking up a CD and a report for the procedures, and hand-carry them with you to your first consultation visit. Do the same with the pathology slides from your biopsy or surgery.

You may wonder why you need to get these films and slides if they have the reports, but accredited cancer centers and consultants will review the images and, most importantly, the pathology slides to verify their accuracy. There have been reviews in which a pathologist who specializes in lymphomas discovers that the pathology is different than initially stated, and that the patient doesn't have lymphoma or has a different kind of lymphoma. Accuracy is critical for pathology. Your treatment plan at every step is based on this information being correct.

LEARNING ABOUT YOUR DISEASE BEFORE THE FIRST VISIT

Lymphoma is cancer of the lymphatic system or, simply put, "cancer of lymph nodes." The lymphatic system is composed of the spleen (an organ located in the upper left abdomen, next to the stomach, that filters blood and helps with immunity) and lymph nodes (small filtering tissues that cleanse fluid that seeps out of the blood vessels). Lymph nodes are comprised of lymphocytes, a type of white blood cell that helps the body fight infection and contributes to the body's immunity. In lymphoma, abnormal lymphocytes begin to grow in a rapid and uncontrolled manner, almost always due to non-inherited genetic mutations. Although we can sometimes attribute this genetic damage to pesticides, radiation exposure, or certain viruses such as the Epstein-Barr virus (which also causes mononucleosis), most of the time there is no known or attributable cause.

While the presence of abnormal and enlarged lymph glands can raise a clinical suspicion of lymphoma, the diagnosis requires pathological confirmation by a biopsy. This involves the removal of an entire lymph node by a surgeon. This procedure is called an excisional biopsy, and it is usually a relatively simple outpatient procedure. Sometimes a needle biopsy ("FNA," or fine needle aspiration) will suffice, especially when the lymph nodes are in hard to reach places. This involves inserting a fine needle into the lymph node and removing cellular tissue (cytology) for examination in the pathology laboratory. If possible, a core biopsy is also done along with the needle biopsy. This involves removing a small piece of the lymph node by inserting a larger biopsy needle into it. In addition to looking at the biopsy material under the microscope, the pathologist will send the tissue samples for several complex laboratory tests: flow cytometry, cytogenetic (chromosomal) analysis and molecular studies. These special tests help the pathologist determine with certainty that the lymph node abnormality is a malignant one, and establish the exact subtype of lymphoma that is present. Accurate diagnosis, prognosis, and management depend on this type of sophisticated testing. Because the diagnosis of lymphoma, particularly its sub-type, can be difficult to make, it is important to have a pathologist with expertise in the diagnosis of lymphoma (a hematopathologist) review the biopsy material and the special tests results.

Lymphoma is broadly classified as either non-Hodgkin's lymphoma (NHL) or Hodgkin's lymphoma (HL, also called Hodgkin's disease). These are described in the next section.

NON-HODGKIN'S LYMPHOMA (NHL)

1. Is it common?

NHL is the most common hematological (blood and lymph node) cancer. Currently, there are almost a half million people in the United States living with NHL (with active disease or in remission). About 65,000 people are diagnosed with NHL every year in the United States. The incidence of lymphoma has been increasing almost every year since the 1980s; part of the increase is most likely due to better detection methods, while another major cause is the aging of our population, because lymphoma incidences increase as people age and their immune systems weaken (see Chapter 10). Although NHL may occur at any age, most cases present after age 50 and are almost equally distributed among males and females, although the exact distribution can vary by sub-type of NHL.

2. What does it mean?

NHL can be considered a "melting pot" of lymphomas. There are at least three dozen different types of NHLs, and researchers continually identify new entities among patients who are currently grouped together. One way to broadly classify these NHL types is to think of them as either indolent or aggressive lymphomas.

3. Which subtype do you have and what is its significance?

Indolent (also called Low-Grade) Lymphoma

Table 1 summarizes the list of indolent lymphomas. These lymphomas are usually very slow growing, presenting without symptoms (fever, night sweats, or weight loss) and with almost stable radiology findings or lymph nodes that wax and wane or even spontaneously disappear. Follicular lymphomas are the most common type of indolent lymphomas and usually occur in multiple sites such as numerous lymph nodes, spleen, and bone marrow. Despite being in so many locations, these lymphomas usually have a long, protracted course, sometimes not even requiring therapy. Indolent lymphomas should be thought of as chronic diseases like diabetes and hypertension: They are incurable (exceptions might occur in localized presentations, which are rare, or after very aggressive therapy such as bone marrow/stem cell transplantation), but many people can live with them for years or even decades with minimal treatment or intermittent treatment.

Table 1   List of Indolent or Low-Grade Lymphomas
(in alphabetical order)

Follicular lymphomas

Hairy cell leukemia

Large granular lymphocytic leukemia (LGL)

Lymphoplasmacytic lymphoma/ Waldenström's
macroglobulinemia

Marginal zone lymphoma
- Extranodal MALT (mucosa-associated lymphoid
tumor) lymphoma
- Nodal marginal zone lymphoma
- Splenic marginal zone lymphoma

Mycosis fungoides /Sézary syndrome

Nodular lymphocyte predominant Hodgkin's lymphoma

Primary cutaneous anaplastic large cell lymphoma/
lymphomatoid papulosis

Small lymphocytic lymphoma /chronic lymphocytic leukemia

The first priority with indolent lymphoma is to decide if watchful waiting without any therapy is an option. Staging studies such as PET (positron emission tomography) or CAT (computed tomography) scans, bone marrow biopsies, patient symptoms, and blood tests help the physician decide whether therapy is essential. Generally, reasons for starting therapy include bulky disease, fever, soaking night sweats, anemia, low white cell count, low platelet count, and liver or kidney damage by the lymphoma.

It should be noted, however, that not everyone has a protracted course with indolent lymphomas. Some patients relapse (i.e., lymphoma comes back despite full treatment) quickly, and sometimes the lymphoma transforms into an aggressive lymphoma.

With many years ahead of them, young patients may face uncertain future prospects. However, lymphoma research is very active, and many new therapies and approaches have been introduced recently. Many more are expected in the near future. Controlling disease can provide time for new treatment to become available. Remember that lymphoma is one of the most responsive conditions to chemotherapy and immunotherapy.

Aggressive (also called High-Grade) Lymphoma

Aggressive or high-grade lymphomas are usually fast growing, often with symptoms such as fevers, night sweats, or weight loss. NHL usually occurs in more than one location, and sometimes involves some of the body's other organs, such as bone marrow, lungs, or liver. The most common type of aggressive lymphoma is diffuse large B cell lymphoma. Treatment with chemotherapy or immunotherapy usually is required quickly. Fortunately, most aggressive lymphomas respond to treatment well and can be cured in a large proportion of patients. Even with subsequent relapse, some patients are still curable with more aggressive treatment involving stem cell transplantation, immunotherapy, or radiation therapy. **Table 2** summarizes the list of aggressive or high-grade lymphomas.

4. What is the treatment?

Watchful waiting is sometimes the best "treatment" for an indolent lymphoma. When treatment is required, it is usually with chemotherapy, but radiation therapy may also have a role in controlling symptoms. Surgery is not used to treat lymphoma. Treatment is discussed in detail in Chapter 3.

Table 2 List of Aggressive or High-Grade Lymphomas (in alphabetical order)

Adult T-cell leukemia/lymphoma

AIDS-related lymphoma

Anaplastic large cell (Ki-1) lymphoma

Angioimmunoblastic T-cell lymphoma

Burkitt's lymphoma/Burkitt's-like lymphoma/ Burkitt's leukemia

Classical Hodgkin's lymphoma

Diffuse large B-cell lymphoma

Extranodal NK/T-cell lymphoma, nasal type

Follicular large B-cell lymphoma

Hepatosplenic gamma/delta T-cell lymphoma

Intravascular large B-cell lymphoma

Lymphomatoid granulomatosis

Mantle cell lymphoma

Peripheral T-cell lymphoma

Post-transplant lymphoproliferative disorder

Precursor B- or T-cell lymphoblastic lymphoma/ leukemia (ALL)

Primary central nervous system (CNS) lymphoma

Primary effusion lymphoma

Primary mediastinal large B-cell lymphoma

Prolymphocytic leukemia

Subcutaneus panniculitis-like T-cell lymphoma

True histiocytic lymphoma

5. What is the prognosis?

The average 5-year survival rate for NHL patients is about 70% overall. This does not mean you would live only 5 years. Rather, it describes the average proportion of people with NHL who are alive after 5 years. Note, this is just an average, and many people live longer than that. Even more importantly, your individual prognosis will vary depending on whether your lymphoma is indolent or aggressive, what the stage of your disease is, and what your response to therapy is.

There are a couple of prognostic tools, such as the International Prognostic Index (IPI), that can predict the prognosis of your lymphoma more accurately. The IPI takes 5 factors to create an estimate of survival for aggressive lymphomas, particularly for the most common type of aggressive lymphoma, diffuse large B-cell lymphoma. These factors include age 60 or over, stage III or IV disease, high lactate dehydrogenase (LDH) levels in the blood, performance status (how fit you are), and 2 or more locations outside of the lymph nodes (in other body organs). The number of these adverse factors can then divide patients into favorable, intermediate, or poor prognostic categories. Fortunately, thanks to breakthroughs such as the use of Rituxan (rituximab) with combination chemotherapy, even patients who start in the poor prognostic group have a better than 50% chance of cure after 5 to 10 years.

A similar prognostic index exists for indolent low-grade lymphomas, particularly for the most common type, follicular lymphomas. This index is called the Follicular Lymphoma International Prognostic Index (FLIPI) and also tabulates the number of risk factors to assess a prognostic group. Even for the worst group of patients, more than 50% of them are alive after 5 years.

You should speak to your physician about the prognosis for your specific lymphoma because individual medical issues will certainly affect these prognostic tools. The greatest value of these groupings is to ensure better conduct of clinical trials and better assessment and comparison of published results. These prognostic scores may not be accurate when making predictions for individuals, but they can be helpful when used as a general guide for treatment choice.

HODGKIN'S LYMPHOMA (HL)

1. Is HL common?

There are more than 150,000 people in the United States living with HL (with active disease or in remission). It is estimated that about 8,000 adults are diagnosed with HL every year. It accounts for about 10% of all lymphomas. HL peaks between the ages of 15 to 35 and again in the elderly (over age 50), but may occur at any age. Younger patients tend to do much better than older patients for any given stage despite similar treatments, suggesting a biologic difference in the disease at different ages.

2. What does it mean?

HL is a lymphoma diagnosed by characteristic "Reed-Sternberg" cells seen microscopically in the pathology biopsy specimen. These cells are large cells with two or more round nodules (nuclei) in the center that give it a characteristic "owl's eye" appearance under the microscope. HL was the first type of lymphoma to be identified by Thomas Hodgkin in the mid-1800s. For this reason all subsequent lymphomas (now numbering more than three dozen) have been called non-Hodgkin's lymphomas.

3. Which subtype do you have and what is its significance?

HL can be further classified into four sub-categories based on the pathological characteristics of the lymphoma: nodular sclerosis Hodgkin's lymphoma (NSHL), mixed cellularity Hodgkin's lymphoma (MCHL), lymphocyte-depleted Hodgkin's lymphoma (LDHL), and lymphocyte-predominant Hodgkin's lymphoma (LPHL). NSHL is the most common subtype of HL in the United States. NSHL, MCHL, and LDHL have similar features and are often classified as classical HL. LPHL, however, is different biologically and clinically and can be considered similar to an indolent or low-grade lymphoma.

4. What is the treatment?

HL is usually treated with chemotherapy, but sometimes radiation therapy is used. This is discussed in detail in Chapter 3.

5. What is the prognosis?

HL generally has a good prognosis. That said, not everyone does well and it would be incorrect to speak of this as a "good" lymphoma. The stage and symptoms are the most important prognostic factors, but other determinants include the erythrocyte sedimentation rate (ESR) of the blood, the number of lymph node or other organ sites involved, and size of the lymph nodes.

Patients with Stage I or II disease (see the following section, Cancer Staging) and no other adverse features are referred to as Early Favorable patients. Generally, these patients do very well with a better than 90% cure rate at 10 years, using either 4 doses of chemotherapy (usually the ABVD regimen described in Chapter 3) plus involved nodal radiation, or with 8 doses of chemotherapy alone.

Patients with Stage I or II disease and any one of the mentioned adverse features are referred to as "Early Unfavorable" patients. These patients have an 85-90% cure rate using 12 doses of chemotherapy (still ABVD) with or without involved node radiation. The use of radiation here is controversial. Any advantage of controlling disease locally with radiation may be offset by long-term side effects from the radiation, including second malignancies and coronary heart disease, which may occur over decades with increasing incidence.

Finally, all patients with stage III or IV disease and those with stage IIB disease (with fever, soaking night sweats, or significant weight loss), are referred to as Advanced patients. A complicated international prognostic score also exists to subdivide advanced patients into a favorable or unfavorable group. These patients usually receive 12 doses of ABVD chemotherapy in the United States, but internationally, other regimens (such as escalated and standard dose BEACOPP) are used for patients with an unfavorable prognosis. Studies are now underway to determine if PET/CAT scans obtained after 4 doses (2 cycles) of chemotherapy can be used to help guide subsequent treatment decisions.

This section only provides rough estimates for HL prognosis, and it is important to factor in new therapies as they evolve; again, it is important to speak with your doctor for your own individualized prognosis.

CANCER STAGING

Let's jump-start your knowledge base a bit before your doctor's visit and review with you the findings from the pathology found on the lymph node biopsy. Initially, all information printed on medical reports and told to you will sound like a foreign language. By the end of your treatment you will be quoting this information yourself with confidence and knowledge. Some people say they could write their own encyclopedia on their disease when they finish treatment. It's probably true. Most biopsies are done as an excisional or core biopsy (see page 4) so that enough tissue can be examined to accurately determine the diagnosis and sub-type of lymphoma. The biopsy and pathological examination of the specimen is a crucial step as it provides information about the type of lymphoma you have, and is one of the most important factors in determining the treatment and prognosis of your lymphoma. Putting together information from your imaging studies along with the biopsy information provides what is needed to determine your staging and subsequent treatment recommendations.

The stage of disease describes the extent of lymphoma in the body. It is a very important factor that determines the type of therapy you will receive and your prognosis. The most common classification is the Ann Arbor staging, which is particularly important for HL:

Stage I. Lymphoma is present in only one region or group of lymph node(s).

Stage II. Lymphoma is present in more than one region or group of lymph nodes but all the groups are on the same side (above or below) of the diaphragm (muscle that divides the chest from the abdomen).

Stage III. Lymphoma is present in more than one region or group of lymph nodes, both above and below the diaphragm.

Stage IV. Lymphoma is present outside of lymph nodes in organs such as bone marrow, spinal cord, and so on.

Each stage is further classified as A or B. If you have symptoms such as fevers, night sweats, or significant weight loss, then you would be classified as having "B" symptoms; otherwise, you would be classified as "A."

Remember:

- Most patients with HL and aggressive NHLs respond to the current chemotherapy regimens, and many are cured of the disease.

- Many patients with indolent lymphomas have long periods of time not requiring therapy, and a watchful waiting policy is optimal. When treatment is required, more than a dozen types of therapies are available to induce a remission and some of these treatments can be reapplied at a later date if initially successful. Use of Rituxan during initial treatment and continued use during maintenance treatment has improved survival and tripled remission durations for the indolent low-grade lymphomas.

- It is natural to feel emotionally upset, so do not hesitate to ask for help.

- The side effects from chemotherapy can be minimized with the use of drugs now available for that purpose.

- Most people work and continue their activities of daily living during treatment.

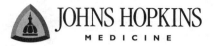

CHAPTER 2

JOHNS HOPKINS
M E D I C I N E

My Team—
Meeting Your
Treatment Team

TEAM MEMBERS—MEDICAL ONCOLOGIST/ HEMATOLOGIST, RADIATION ONCOLOGIST, RADIOLOGIST, PATHOLOGIST, NURSES, AND OTHERS

There will be many people on your oncology team helping you to be well again. Each has a specific role and specialty related to lymphoma and its treatment. The following is a list of the major players:

Medical Hematologist, Oncologist, or Hematologist/Oncologist. This is a physician who selects medicines for systemic treatment that may include chemotherapy and/or targeted immunotherapy. This doctor is usually consulted after your diagnosis of lymphoma has been confirmed (nurse practitioners and physician assistants can provide excellent care and dedicate extra time for you in the initial stages of your diagnosis).

Radiation Oncologist. This physician specializes in using forms of radiation therapy.

Radiologist. This doctor may have performed the CAT scan as well as the core biopsy to diagnose you. Additional radiological imaging studies may be done by this physician as well.

Pathologist. Though you will probably never meet this person, he or she is one of the most important people on your team. The pathologist looks under the microscope at your biopsy tissue and your lymphoma surgery tissue to determine the type of lymphoma and provides important prognostic information that is used to determine your treatment plan.

Nurses. There will be several nurses involved with your care. You will probably meet a new one at each stage of your treatment, beginning with surgery, then chemotherapy, then radiation, and finally long-term care. They are responsible for providing patient education, assessing your clinical needs, administering chemotherapy drugs, and evaluating your progress during treatment.

Social Worker. This degreed and licensed professional helps coordinate any personal needs you might have, from assisting with financial issues to arranging for home health care (if necessary) to linking you with support systems and other networks.

Survivor Volunteer. Many cancer centers and practices offer emotional support through survivor volunteers who have completed their treatment of lymphoma and want to provide one-on-one support to newly diagnosed lymphoma patients such as yourself. They provide a candid view of what to expect and can be great support along your journey.

MAKING YOUR INITIAL APPOINTMENT

Initially, you will meet with a medical oncologist and/or hematologist about your lymphoma diagnosis. This doctor specializes in the field of chemotherapy and treats lymphoma. There are many doctors who call themselves lymphoma specialists. That doesn't mean they are specialists or were trained as such. It is useful to know their credentials, board certification, and the volume of lymphoma patients they treat, and to ask them about outcomes or quality measures. You have the right to get these answers. If the doctor says he or she does not know, that may be a signal for you to seek guidance and treatment elsewhere. All physicians know the volume of lymphoma patients they treat. It's not a mystery.

Be sure that the intake person helping to arrange your appointment knows that you are newly diagnosed with lymphoma. Most facilities arrange for patient appointments quite promptly. Symptomatic patients should be seen promptly, but most patients will not suffer from a delay of several days or even a few weeks. However, a longer delay of more than a month is generally not advisable as some of the lymphomas can be aggressive and potentially lethal if not treated soon. Rapid lymph node growth, the presence of symptoms, or markedly abnormal laboratory tests usually mandate a fast evaluation and start of therapy. Slowly growing disease often found incidentally, with few symptoms and few abnormal laboratory tests, does not require a fast evaluation. Aggressive lymphomas are more worrisome, while indolent lymphomas are not as worrisome, even in advanced stage, because a watchful waiting approach may be the best option.

Be sure to get a specific address and clear directions for where you are to go and what time you are to report there. If you haven't been to this facility before, allow yourself extra drive time to find it, find parking, and get to the location. Being late only frustrates you more and your doctor as well. Arriving early gives you time to sit in the waiting area and review your questions one more time so your visit is as productive as possible.

You've got your appointment and directions for where to go and what time to arrive. More than likely the scheduler with whom you spoke also provided you instructions regarding what to bring. Just in case the information wasn't clear, we provide the following to help ensure that your visit is as productive and efficient as possible for you and the doctor who will be seeing you.

WHAT TO BRING WITH YOU FOR THAT FIRST CONSULTATION

It's time for your first consultation with a qualified medical oncologist and/or hematologist. Bring with you pertinent records, radiologic studies (usually PETs/CTs), and pathology reports. The doctor may have requested that the pathology slides be shipped in advance so that his or her own pathologist can look at them before your arrival and render an opinion about the accuracy of the information provided in the original biopsy report. Also know in advance if your insurance company requires you to get preauthorization for having additional tests done. There are situations in which the doctor reviews the films and finds them less than satisfactory. When this occurs, he or she may want to get additional imaging done while you are there for this visit. Your doctor may ask that you leave your CTs and other imaging studies there for him or her to show to others too (such as colleagues or at a tumor board/conference). You may have been told by the facility where they were originally done that you must bring them back right away. Not so. These images are technically your property. The doctor needs to retain them for a time and will use them during your medical care. So don't feel intimidated if the facility where they were done makes demands on you that your doctor says you cannot fulfill. Leave it to his or her office to handle any questions/inquiries about when the x-rays will be returned.

WHO TO BRING WITH YOU

Bring a trusted family member or friend with you. When someone is stressed he or she only hears and retains a small portion of what is said. The doctor will be providing a lot of information, and you may feel overwhelmed trying to keep it all straight in your mind. The person with you can serve as a scribe so you can remember important points. It also can be helpful to bring a tape recorder with you. Most doctors are very comfortable with the discussion being voice recorded. Encourage your guest to ask questions as well.

WHAT ELSE TO BRING

Be sure to bring an accurate list of what medical problems you have previously had; what medications you are taking, including vitamins and herbs; what allergies you might have; and your family history for cancers, heart disease, diabetes, lung disease, and other serious illnesses. If you aren't sure, call another family member and recruit help in obtaining this information because it is important for your medical summary and may influence some decision making about your treatment recommendations.

WHAT QUESTIONS TO ASK DURING YOUR VISIT

Having a list of questions prepared in advance is helpful in making the time you have with the doctor as efficient and optimal as possible. The following list will help you get started:

1. What type of lymphoma do I have?

2. What stage of disease do you estimate I have based on what you know so far from my clinical examination and from radiological tests done thus far?

3. Did your pathology team here confirm the accuracy of the biopsy results?

4. Will I need additional tests?

5. What are the treatment options?

6. When will the treatment start?

7. How long will the treatment last?

8. What educational information do you offer to prepare me for chemotherapy and what to expect in terms of side effects?

9. May I speak to a lymphoma survivor volunteer who had a similar treatment plan to what you plan for me?

10. Who will be my contact here for questions I may have?

11. Do you have educational materials for other family members, such as my children?

12. How many lymphoma patients do you see in a year?

13. Who else will be involved in my care and when will I meet them?

14. How often will I see you during the treatment?

15. Are there any clinical trials that you would want to recommend for me to consider at this point?

16. Who will be coordinating my care? Do you have a patient navigator?

17. How are subsequent appointments arranged for me and when do these happen?

WHAT TESTS NEED TO BE DONE

You most likely received the diagnosis of lymphoma after the pathologist reviewed the biopsy slides and confirmed that the pathological features are consistent with this diagnosis. Now, before the treatment can be started, a few investigations are needed to stage disease and decide on the best and safest treatment:

1. *Blood tests.* These tests usually involve the following panel:

    a. Complete blood count, or CBC, evaluates the capacity of your body to make red cells or hemoglobin (blood cells involved in carrying oxygen in the blood to various organs), white cells (blood cells involved in fighting infection), and platelets (blood cells involved in preventing bleeding after a cut).

    b. Comprehensive metabolic panel evaluates kidney function, liver function, and electrolytes, so that the dose of chemotherapy can be calculated correctly and given safely.

c. Hepatitis B virus, hepatitis C virus, and HIV serologies evaluate the presence of these viruses because they can be associated with lymphoma.

d. Lactate dehydrogenase, or LDH, can serve as a tumor marker (another marker of response) under some circumstances. However, LDH can be increased under various conditions that are unrelated to lymphoma, so speak to your physician about the significance and interpretation of high LDH for your lymphoma.

2. *Radiological investigations.* These usually involve the following scans:

a. A CAT, or computed tomography, is often used in conjunction with a PET. A CAT scanner is a "fancy X-ray" machine that takes pictures of various slices of your body that are later combined to identify abnormal/enlarged lymph nodes. This helps the physician identify the extent of disease and stage of HL (see staging in Chapter 1 for classification).

b. A PET, or positron emission tomography, is often combined with a CAT. PET is a functional scan. A special radioactive glucose is injected in the vein and the amount of glucose taken by various tissues is analyzed by a special camera. Cancer cells divide rapidly and need more glucose than normal tissues. Thus they light up more (or are more "hot") than normal tissues, and this is used to evaluate the extent of disease.

3. *Bone marrow biopsy.* In certain instances (depending on the stage of disease and the results of the PET/CAT), your physician might recommend a bone

marrow biopsy. This procedure, as the name suggests, requires inserting a small biopsy needle through the bone into the bone marrow (space in the bone involved in the production of blood cells). The biopsy site is usually in the back of your hipbone. The biopsy is usually done as an outpatient, in your hematologist/oncologist's office. Although you may experience some discomfort with the procedure, most people are able to tolerate the procedure well with generous amounts of local anesthesia. However, if you are worried about pain or if you had a bad experience with a previous bone marrow biopsy, the procedure could be done under sedation (putting you to sleep) and you should speak to your physician about it.

4. *Echocardiogram or MUGA (multiple-gated acquisition) scan.* These tests image the heart and provide information regarding its structure and function. One of the chemotherapy agents (Adriamycin [doxorubicin]) could affect the function of the heart in a small proportion of patients, and thus a baseline test is obtained before starting chemotherapy.

5. *Lumbar puncture.* In certain instances (depending on the type and stage of NHL), your physician may recommend a lumbar puncture or spinal tap. This is an outpatient procedure that is done to obtain cerebrospinal fluid to assess whether there is lymphoma involvement in the brain and spinal cord. A needle is inserted into the back and spinal fluid is obtained. This is then examined under the microscope to look for presence of lymphoma cells. Sometimes chemotherapy is also given into the spine (called "intrathecal chemotherapy") to kill lymphoma cells in the brain and spinal cord.

HOW BEST TO CONTACT TEAM MEMBERS

Request business cards from each healthcare provider you see and ask what their office procedure is for responding to questions/concerns you may have. Usually, there is one contact person who serves in this role. Also find out if you are at liberty to communicate with any of the team by e-mail. If and when the need arises and you have questions, be succinct and think all your thoughts through. It's better to ask three questions at once than one question three different times in a row.

NAVIGATING APPOINTMENTS

Some cancer centers or large practices have patient navigators. However, the term "navigation" is loosely defined and in some cases is used for simply marketing and not truly to navigate someone along his or her journey. When you inquire about this, ask about the process for assisting you with appointment scheduling, getting test results, getting scheduled for your chemotherapy, seeing the medical oncologist emergently, and being available in general for support and to address any other clinical needs that may arise. In some cases your point person may be a nurse or an office manager in the doctor's office. In other cases it may be someone who is called a navigator or case manager. Their title isn't as important as their functions.

FINANCIAL IMPLICATIONS OF TREATMENT/ INSURANCE CLEARANCE

You didn't plan on getting diagnosed with lymphoma right now. No doubt this was never one of your goals. There is no convenient time to get this disease, and the diagnosis alone can raise havoc in your life. If you work outside the home, you will be taking time off for your chemotherapy, at least for the first couple of cycles and possibly for the whole duration of chemotherapy. Getting your ducks in a row early on is smart. Finding out about sick leave, short-term disability coverage, copayment information, prescription coverage, and other medical expense issues is helpful for planning your budget. Your insurance company may require referrals to see certain specialists, to have tests done, or to get chemotherapy or other treatments authorized. If you need help with these things, ask for a social worker to assist you. In some cases, cancer centers have financial assistants for this purpose.

Some recommended treatments may relate to clinical trials. Some may be covered by your insurance, and others may not. If participating in a clinical trial, a research nurse will assist with getting this type of information answered for you.

If you lack health insurance, all is not lost. There are resources available for people who need help and meet certain criteria for financial assistance and coverage of their lymphoma treatment expenses. Some states even have special grants for residents for precisely this purpose. Check with the social worker at the facility where you are being treated to get assistance and referrals. There are also organizations that provide support for transportation to and from treatment visits, provide food for you and your family, and even assist with coverage of some medications. They aren't available in every state so you will have to rely on the social worker to tell you more about what is available in your geographic area.

Financial support services are not well advertised. It will require you to take the initiative to ask about them rather than waiting for someone to tell you about them. Be assertive and do this for yourself. That's why these programs exist. Money is the primary reason family members get into arguments. Avoid this up front by discussing the issue and planning a budget. Be proactive in asking to meet with the social worker to discuss what support services are available for you as well.

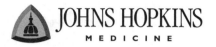

CHAPTER 3

TAKING ACTION— COMPREHENSIVE TREATMENT CONSIDERATIONS

Lymphoma treatment generally includes chemotherapy or immunotherapy, and sometimes radiation therapy, surgery, or stem cell transplantation. Some patients need all these therapies; others just need one. The number of therapies doesn't always match up with the severity of the disease. Let's review each one.

CHEMOTHERAPY AND/OR TARGETED IMMUNOTHERAPY

Chemotherapy and/or targeted immunotherapy are the cornerstone of therapy for most lymphomas, except for a few early-stage lymphomas.

Chemotherapy is based on the concept of killing dividing cells. Because lymphoma cells divide rapidly, chemotherapy blocks their division and kills them. Chemotherapy is a systemic therapy that is infused or injected into the bloodstream through the vein and has the potential to kill cancer cells wherever they are. Having said that, normal cells in the body also divide, particularly in the gastrointestinal tract and bone marrow, and chemotherapy may also kill those cells. Thus you may experience side effects such as hair loss, nausea, vomiting, diarrhea, and a drop in blood cell counts. The good thing is that these side effects are mostly reversible and diminish once the chemotherapy cycles are complete.

In recent years targeted immunotherapies, particularly monoclonal antibodies, have been developed. These monoclonal antibodies bind to specific receptors that are present in larger numbers on cancer cells and less so on normal cells, and thus selectively kill cancer cells.

A simple way to understand this is to consider chemotherapy as a "grenade" that can effectively destroy the enemy house but can cause collateral damage (side effects). Targeted immunotherapies are like sharp-shooting rifles that selectively kill enemies but might not be able to kill the enemy if it is hidden (the receptor is not expressed).

Chemotherapy and/or immunotherapy are most commonly administered into the bloodstream through the vein. It can often be given in an outpatient setting. However, for the most aggressive lymphomas (like Burkitt's lymphoma), intensive chemotherapy is needed that is often best delivered in the hospital setting. Some people have "difficult" veins to puncture in the arm, and chemotherapy can scar the veins and make them difficult to use. A long-term intravenous catheter like a Hickman catheter or a Port-A-Cath or PICC (peripherally inserted central catheter) is often placed to overcome these difficulties and establish long term access for the duration of chemotherapy. Ask your physician whether these catheters would be advisable for you.

There are various chemotherapy regimens (treatment programs). Chemotherapy is generally given in cycles. Each cycle is usually 21–28 days long. Do not fear that you will get chemotherapy on all these days. Generally, chemotherapy is given on day 1 and then the intervening days allow for the chemotherapy to work and for the body to recover from the side effects of chemotherapy. Blood is checked in between (usually once a week) to ensure that the liver, kidney, and bone marrow functions are within expected ranges. The same chemotherapy is then repeated (usually after 14–21 days) during the next cycle.

A repeat CAT is usually obtained after two or three cycles to ensure the lymphoma is shrinking. The use of PET or PET/CAT scans in this situation is controversial and is currently the subject of clinical investigations. When the PET/CAT shows substantial shrinkage after two to three cycles, this is usually a very favorable sign. However, sometimes scans may be falsely positive, i.e., they may show an abnormality that is not cancer. Any change in therapy might be dangerous or unnecessary in this situation until we understand how to better confirm the need for switching treatment.

When the repeat CAT scan after two to three cycles shows significant improvement, the same chemotherapy is continued for a few more cycles. If the lymphoma is not shrinking, that suggests the lymphoma is not responding to the current chemotherapy regimen and an alternate regimen and/or stem cell transplant (later in this chapter) should be considered.

On average, a total of six chemotherapy cycles are given. Some patients may get four and some may get eight cycles depending on the type of lymphoma, the stage, the response to therapy, and physician preference. Sometimes for follicular NHL, after the initial combination chemotherapy is over, maintenance immunotherapy with an antibody called Rituxan is given (every 2–3 months or for 4 consecutive weeks every 6 months for about 2 years, and sometimes longer).

The treatment regimens for NHL and HL are different. Typical regimens used for new patients are discussed in the next section. However, your physician may recommend a different regimen depending on the stage and type of NHL or HL. The following information is meant to serve as a general guide.

NON-HODGKIN'S LYMPHOMA (NHL)

Although there are various chemotherapy regimens for NHL, one of the most common regimens used currently is R-CHOP (Rituxan, Cytoxan [cyclophosphamide], hydroxydoxorubicin, Oncovin [vincristine], and prednisone).

Other common NHL regimens include Rituxan alone (especially for indolent low-grade lymphomas); R-CVP (Rituxan, Cytoxan, vincristine, and prednisone); FCR (fludarabine, Cytoxan, and Rituxan); R-EPOCH (Rituxan, etoposide, prednisone, Oncovin, Cytoxan, hydroxydoxorubicin), which is usually given as an inpatient procedure; and R-ICE (Rituxan, Ifex (ifosfamide), carboplatin, and etoposide).

HODGKIN'S LYMPHOMA (HL)

There are various chemotherapy regimens for HL. One of the most common regimens used currently is ABVD (Adriamycin, bleomycin, vinblastine, and dacarbazine).

CHEMOTHERAPY AGENTS

A brief description of each chemotherapy agent follows (listed alphabetically):

Adriamycin is an intravenous chemotherapy drug that interferes with DNA (the genetic material controlling cell growth and division) and blocks cell growth. Common side effects include hair loss, nausea, and drop in blood counts. It can be toxic to the liver and heart. The latter is usually seen after the cumulative dose of Adriamycin exceeds 500 mg/m2 (i.e., after 10 doses). Your physician will check weekly blood counts and kidney and liver function to monitor for these side effects. An echocardiogram is usually obtained at baseline and sometimes after the end of six cycles to monitor the function of the heart. If you notice the presence of shortness of breath with exertion (even years after chemotherapy), speak to your physician because this could be a sign of cardiomyopathy (heart dysfunction), a late side effect of Adriamycin.

Bleomycin is an intravenous chemotherapy drug that causes DNA damage and stops cell growth. Common side effects include hair loss, nausea, and drop in blood counts. If you notice the presence of shortness of breath or increasing cough (even years after chemotherapy), speak to your physician because this could be a sign of pulmonary toxicity (lung damage), a known side effect of bleomycin. Most physicians order pulmonary function tests before using this drug and after every two to three doses to monitor for bleomycin-induced lung damage.

Cytoxan is an intravenous chemotherapy drug that damages DNA and results in cell death. Common side effects include hair loss, nausea, and drop in blood counts. It can be toxic to the kidneys and the urinary bladder, and this can be minimized by keeping the body well hydrated and ensuring you have a good urine output. Your physician will check weekly blood counts and kidney and liver function in between cycles to monitor for these side effects. If you notice the presence of red urine, speak to your physician because this could be a sign of hemorrhagic cystitis (inflammation of the urinary bladder), a rare, late side effect of Cytoxan.

Dacarbazine is an intravenous chemotherapy. Common side effects include allergic reaction, nausea, diarrhea, and lowering of blood counts.

Oncovin, more commonly known by its generic name vincristine, is an intravenous chemotherapy drug. Unlike other chemotherapy agents, it can actually cause constipation rather than diarrhea. If you notice the presence of weakness in your arms or legs or any numbness or tingling sensation, speak to your physician because this could be a sign of peripheral neuropathy (damage to nerves), a known side effect of vincristine.

Prednisone is a type of corticosteroid that is given orally for 5 days with chemotherapy. Although it is not a chemotherapy agent per se, it augments the efficacy of chemotherapy agents. It is also a good antinausea medication. Side effects are minimal in the short term but could include weight gain, stomach ulcer (taking an acid suppressant is a good idea), temporary increases in blood sugar, bone loss, visual disturbance, and mood swings. Insomnia is a common side effect while on steroids, and short-acting sleeping pills may be required.

Rituxan is an intravenous monoclonal antibody/targeted therapy against the CD20 receptor that is expressed on lymphoma cells. It is generally well tolerated. Side effects include infusion-related reactions such as chills and shaking (rigors) that can be minimized by slowing the rate of Rituxan infusion and by using premedications such as Tylenol (acetaminophen), Benadryl (diphenhydramine), and dexamethasone (a steroid) intravenously. Over time, Rituxan may suppress the immune system and increase the risk of infections.

Vinblastine and vincristine are sister intravenous chemotherapy drugs, derived from the *Vinca* plant genus. Unlike other chemotherapy agents, these can actually cause constipation rather than diarrhea. If you notice the presence of weakness in your arms or legs or any sensory disturbance, speak to your physician because this could be a sign of peripheral neuropathy (damage to nerves), a known side effect of these drugs.

RADIATION THERAPY

Radiation therapy is sometimes used for early-stage lymphomas, before or after chemotherapy. Radiation therapy is also used in special cases such as spinal cord compression or for extra-large masses (>10 cm). Radiation can also be attached to a targeted monoclonal antibody to deliver treatment directly to the lymphoma cells.

SURGERY

Surgery alone is generally not used to treat lymphoma, except when an excisional lymph node biopsy is required or when invasive surgery is required to establish a diagnosis. Sometimes an enlarged spleen must be removed when other diagnostic tests are unhelpful.

BONE MARROW OR STEM CELL TRANSPLANT

Some lymphomas are resistant to standard treatment or may recur after therapy. In such instances, stem cell transplant (also called bone marrow transplant) is often considered. Stem cell transplantation is a complex procedure that requires a multidisciplinary team of physicians, nurses, social workers, and ancillary staff. It requires meticulous planning, and is typically done in tertiary centers. There are 2 types of stem cell transplant. An autologous stem cell transplant uses cells provided from the patient, whereas allogenic transplants use cells from a family member or a tissue typed unrelated donor

In both autologous and allogeneic transplants very high doses of chemotherapy are used to kill the lymphoma cells. The dose of chemotherapy is so high that it also kills the normal bone marrow (or stem cells). The stem cells that are harvested from the patient (autologous) or donor (allogeneic) are used to rescue the patient's normal bone marrow by replanting it with stem cells so that it will function normally. Allogeneic transplant also produces an immunologic effect that works to kill the lymphoma cells.

Given the complexities, and importance of careful monitoring, most patients require hospitalization for about a month for the procedure, and close follow up afterwards. Because the whole procedure can appear particularly overwhelming, most hospitals have a video/teaching session to educate patients and their families about the procedure and allay any concerns. Please refer to *100 Questions & Answers about Bone Marrow and Stem Cell Transplantation* by Ewa Carrier, MD, MHS and Gracy Ledingham for more details on stem cell transplants.

WATCHFUL WAITING

For many patients with indolent or low-grade lymphomas, not undergoing therapy is an acceptable option because tumors might spontaneously shrink or grow at such a slow rate they would not cause any significant problem, even for years. This decision is based on the sub-type and stage of lymphoma, and can be a difficult one. This option is often under-used due to a fear of "doing nothing for the lymphoma" among patients, family members, and even physicians. However, it should be noted that chemotherapy can have significant side effects, can impair the quality of life, and for some lymphomas such as indolent NHLs, may not be very effective. So, the decision to use chemotherapy should be carefully weighed, and chemotherapy should not be used when it is felt that the adverse effects of the treatment would outweigh any potential benefits.

In general, all patients with indolent low-grade lymphomas, regardless of stage, should be considered for watchful waiting if they meet the following criteria:

1. No constitutional symptoms—no fever, recurrent soaking night sweats, or significant weight loss (greater than 10% baseline weight within 6 months).

2. No abnormally low or high blood counts—no significant anemia (low red blood cells with hemoglobin less than 10 mg/dl), no leukopenia (low white blood cell count at less than 1000 neutrophils/mm³), no thrombocytopenia (low platelet count less than 50,000/mm³) or excessive leukocytosis (high white blood cell count at greater than 200,000/mm³).

3. No impairment of liver or kidney function (by blood tests and/or CAT scans). No hypercalemia (high

calcium level), which invariably means an underlying aggressive lymphoma that requires treatment.

4. No excessively bulky disease that is causing symptoms such as shortness of breath, abdominal fullness, or lack of appetite. This is usually greater than 10 cm in size.

5. Lack of rapid growth of lymph nodes or change in blood counts (with a doubling in 2–4 months).

6. No psychological problems regarding watchful waiting: some patients simply cannot abide the concept of "doing nothing" despite every reassurance.

It is important to be aware of the biases that may discourage a watchful waiting approach. Relatives and friends are often shocked if treatment is not recommended and may push you to get it. Some doctors make more money from treatment than from watching, and others may be motivated to sign up patients for clinical treatment trials. Clinical trials are an important option that you may want to consider, but most indolent low-grade lymphoma studies only accept patients who meet the criteria for treatment outlined above. Genetic factors (which are the wave of the future) are not ready for use at present to inform us whether to consider watchful waiting or to proceed with treatment.

OTHER MEDICATIONS AND INTERVENTIONS (SUPPORTIVE CARE)

ANTIBIOTICS

If you receive chemotherapy, you are more predisposed to have recurrence of herpes/zoster (shingles) infection, and prophylactic antiherpes medication, such as acyclovir, Valtrex (valacyclovir), or Famvir (famciclovir), is often given for the duration of chemotherapy. Another infection that can get reactivated is *Pneumocystis carinii/jiroveci* pneumonia), especially with steroids, and prophylactic anti-*P. carinii/jiroveci* pneumonia medication such as Bactrim (trimethoprim-sulfa) or dapsone is often given for the duration of chemotherapy.

Chemotherapy can lower your white blood cell count, particularly neutrophils (white blood cells involved in fighting infections), and thus lower your body's ability to fight infections. This risk is particularly high when the neutrophil count in your blood is less than 500, which usually occurs between day 7 and 15 of receiving chemotherapy. In this circumstance your physician might prescribe a prophylactic antibiotic, such as a quinolone antibiotic, to help your body fight off an impending infection. If you notice the presence of fever (higher than 99.9 degrees F), you should notify your health team immediately. An infection while you are receiving chemotherapy could be potentially dangerous because your body might not be able to fight it off.

GROWTH FACTOR SUPPORT

As mentioned previously, lymphoma and the chemotherapy used to treat it can lower your white blood cell count, especially neutrophils, lowering your body's ability to fight infections. At times, medications can be used to stimulate a growth factor hormone called granulocyte colony-stimulating factor and help the neutrophils recover faster. Examples include Neupogen (filgrastim), which is given subcutaneously for 10–12 days after chemotherapy, and Neulasta (peg-filgrastim), which is given subcutaneously once on the day after chemotherapy.

ANTINAUSEA MEDICATIONS

One of the most feared side effects of chemotherapy is nausea and vomiting. Fortunately, due to significant research advances in the past couple of decades, nausea and vomiting are better managed now in most instances. You will receive intravenous or oral antinausea medications with your chemotherapy. Depending on the chemotherapy regimen and how you feel, for the next 3–5 days after chemotherapy, when the nausea side effects are at their peak, you may also regularly take other antinausea medications (Zofran [ondansetron] or Anzemet [dolasetron]). If you have nausea/vomiting despite these medications, then you should take breakthrough nausea medications (such as Compazine [prochlorperazine]) prescribed by your physician.

WIGS

Most chemotherapy regimens for lymphoma cause hair loss during treatment. Preparing in advance for this is helpful. This experience can be very traumatic. Seeing someone completely bald, especially women, can imply that we are looking at someone "with cancer." Suggestions for managing hair loss follow:

- Have a hair stylist cut your hair short within two weeks after your first chemotherapy treatment. (This is usually several days before your hair begins falling out).

- Have a "coming out" party for your hair—everyone brings a hat or other head covering (scarf, turban, etc.) This is a great project for children to do for you and helps engage family members in the preparation. Consider it similar to a baby shower, but instead the baby is your head.

- If you plan to wear a wig, get fitted before starting chemotherapy. Take a trusted friend or family member along to give honest feedback regarding how you look. Matching your hair color and style is easier if you go before chemotherapy starts. (There are some patients who opt to have a different hair color and style, because this is an opportunity for a "new look.")

- Some patients choose to have a buzz cut in advance of hair loss, truly taking control of this situation. They don't want the chemotherapy to control when their hair is gone; they will determine its fate. Wearing a baseball cap, hat, turban, or scarf is also an option, as is just plain being bald. It is your choice. During the winter months, however, do wear knitted caps while outdoors or exposed to the elements. We lose significant amounts of body heat from the top of our head. You need to stay bundled up and warm.

- Some insurance companies cover the expenses for a wig, up to a certain amount (usually around $350). It should be submitted on a prescription as a "scalp prosthesis for chemotherapy-induced alopecia" by your medical oncologist, so inquire about this.

CLINICAL TRIALS

Researchers are constantly looking at methods to improve the current management of lymphomas. Clinical trials involve testing of these novel, exciting, but "yet to be proven" ideas. New and innovative treatments are developed and implemented by doing clinical trials. Without clinical trials we could neither improve the treatment of lymphoma nor develop ways to prevent it in the future. Clinical trials form the backbone of science today. Your doctors may at any given time during your treatment discuss with you opportunities to participate in a clinical trial. Be open-minded. Hear what is being offered as part of a study. Let's begin by educating you about clinical trials.

There are many different kinds of clinical trials. They range from studies focusing on ways to prevent, detect, diagnose, treat, or control lymphoma to studies that address quality of life issues that affect our patients. Most clinical trials are carried out in phases. Each phase is designed to learn different information and build on the information previously discovered. Patients may be eligible for studies in different phases depending on their stage of disease, therapies anticipated, as well as treatment they have already had. Patients are monitored at specific intervals while participating in studies too.

> *Phase I studies* determine the best way to do a new treatment and how much of it can be given safely. In such studies only a small number of patients are asked to participate. They are offered to patients whose cancer cannot be helped by other known treatment modalities. These patients are battling end-stage lymphoma and have usually exhausted other treatment options. Some patients personally receive benefit from participation, but others experience no benefit in fighting their cancer. They are, however, paving the way for the next generation, which is important. Once the optimal dose is chosen, the drug is studied for its ability to shrink tumors in phase II trials.

> *Phase II studies* are designed to find out if the treatment actually kills cancer cells in patients. A slightly larger number of patients is selected for this type of trial, usually between 20 and 50 subjects. Patients whose lymphoma has no longer responded to other known treatments may be offered participation in

this type of trial. Tumor shrinkage is measured, and patients are closely observed to measure the effects the treatment is having on treating their disease. Response rates and side effects are also closely monitored and carefully recorded and addressed.

Phase III studies usually compare standard treatments already in use with treatments that appeared to do well in phase II trials. For statistical reasons the study design requires large numbers of patients to participate. Patients are usually randomized for the treatment regimen they will be receiving. These studies are seeking benefits of longer survival, better quality of life, fewer side effects, and fewer cases of cancer recurrence. This is the most common type of clinical trial offered to patients that you may be hearing about.

The following list of questions may help guide you in the decision making and fact finding about clinical trials:

What is the purpose of the study?

How many people will be included in the study?

What does the study involve? What kind of tests and treatment will I have?

How are treatments given and what side effects might I expect?

What are the risks and benefits of each protocol?

How long will the study last?

What type of long-term follow-up care is provided for those who participate?

Will I incur any costs? Will my insurance company pay for part of this?

When will the results be known?

You should appreciate the potential to derive substantial benefit from participating in clinical trials. The current established therapies for lymphomas were in clinical trials a few years ago and are now considered standard therapies after they were found to be effective. Thus the potential advantage of joining a clinical trial is that you would be one of the first to receive these therapies that might be better than the current standard. You would also benefit humankind by furthering science and the understanding of disease. So, be open-minded and discuss potential risks and benefits with your physician as outlined above.

GENERAL TIPS

- Focus on what chemotherapy and/or immunotherapy is designed to do for you—destroy or impede lymphoma cells wherever they occur.

- Most patients feel well the day of the treatment. If side effects occur, they most commonly happen the night of chemotherapy or the next day. Celebrate the completing of each cycle of treatment. Remember you are climbing further up the survival curve by taking treatments. Take pride in this victory. It's important to realize that some patients may react differently to chemotherapy than others. Talking with other lymphoma survivors who have had the same chemotherapy drugs will not really answer the question for you in advance how you personally are going to feel and what side effects you may or may not experience.

- Don't select your treatment regimen based on which drugs do or don't cause hair loss. You want to take the advice of your doctor in helping to decide which drugs will be the right ones for you. You may have several treatment regimens from which to choose. Patients and families naturally want to know which regimen would work best. Your medical oncologist will review your drug options with you based on the prognostic factors learned from your pathology as well as from any scans done in advance of starting your treatment.

- After receiving chemotherapy and/or immunotherapy, your blood will be taken at designated intervals to make sure that your red blood cells and white blood cells are staying within normal limits. If they are low, which is a common side effect, the doctor might decide to give you special medicines to boost your blood counts back up to a normal range.

- Be careful exposing yourself to people who have a cold or flu because your immune system is being taxed right now. Be especially watchful of little children who look healthy but may be little germ carriers.

- Most people today continue to work while receiving chemotherapy. Some patients opt to receive chemotherapy on a Friday and then rest up over the weekend with the help of family and friends.

- Remember, too, that there is a beginning and an end to taking any treatment regimen. We can deal with anything when we know it is for a designated period of time! Positive attitude is the key!

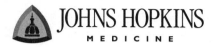

CHAPTER 4

Be Prepared—The Side Effects of Treatment

A patient may experience various side effects while receiving treatment for lymphoma. Some are easily controlled, whereas others may be more difficult. No two patients are alike, so don't assume that if you knew someone with Hodgkin's or non-Hodgkin's lymphoma in the past your situation will mirror his or hers. In this chapter we discuss some of the more common side effects. However, you should also discuss side effects with your oncology team so you have a "head's up" about what to expect in addition to the status of your disease and the treatment recommendations they are making on your behalf. This list can look overwhelming. It is not intended to alarm you, but to provide you with a thorough and comprehensive list of possible issues that may need to be addressed while undergoing treatment.

RITUXAN

This immunological treatment is a cornerstone of therapy for most indolent and aggressive NHLs. Side effects are usually mild in comparison to standard chemotherapeutic drugs. Allergic reactions are the most common side effect and can range from skin rash, shaking chills, fever, and even serious drops in blood pressure with fainting. These reactions usually occur only in the first few infusions, because the body does get used to this medication over time.

Allergic reactions are avoided by taking two Tylenol orally (650 mg) before the infusion and by receiving Benadryl (an antihistamine) and dexamethasone (a corticosteroid) before the Rituxan is administered. In fact, these premedications can cause side effects themselves, such as sedation from the Benadryl during the 4-hour infusion of Rituxan or insomnia at night from the dexamethasone (a sleeping medication may be of help for the insomnia, which rarely lasts more than 48 hours). Reactions can also be avoided by drinking lots of fluids before administration of Rituxan, and intravenous fluids can be supplemented during the infusion if medically allowed. Longer term side effects include lowering of the blood counts and some suppression of the normal immune system, leading to increased risk of infection. However, this usually occurs only after extensive use of Rituxan over years and can be helped by infusions of intravenous immunoglobulin and by stopping the drug.

NAUSEA AND VOMITING

This was once a relatively common side effect associated with administration of some chemotherapy drugs. However, with the development of newer anti-nausea medicines (called antiemetics), the incidence of nausea and vomiting has been reduced considerably and is now experienced by only a few individuals. These medications are usually started before the chemotherapy is administered, either orally or intravenously. The important point is to treat for nausea proactively; it is much easier to control nausea with medication before it occurs. Pain medications have a reputation for contributing to nausea too. If nausea is severe and restricts your ability to eat or retain liquids, dehydration can result. Changing what you eat and drink may also be useful in managing nausea and vomiting. Some specific suggestions are as follows:

Eat a light meal before each chemotherapy treatment.

Eat small amounts of food and liquids at a time.

Eat bland foods and liquids.

Eat dry crackers when feeling nauseated.

Limit the amount of liquids you take with your meals.

Maintain adequate liquids in between meals; take mostly clear liquids such as water, apple juice, herbal tea, or bouillon.

Eat cool foods or foods at room temperature.

Avoid foods with strong odors.

Avoid high-fat, greasy, and fried foods.

Avoid spicy foods, alcohol, and caffeine.

Suck on peppermint candies as an additional way to help reduce or prevent nausea.

Rub peppermint-flavored lip balm above your lip and below your nose so you are smelling mint as a way to also reduce nausea.

Ask your oncologist for a prescription for an antiemetic and ask if you can take it in a preventative manner to reduce and control nausea from happening.

Taking ginger orally or inhaling the aroma nasally can alleviate nausea for some patients.

Motion-sickness wrist bands can be helpful.

Fresh, refrigerated pineapple chunks can remove the metallic taste from drugs such as Cytoxan and may also alleviate nausea or help with a dry mouth.

HAIR LOSS

The technical term is alopecia, but the term patients recognize most clearly is exactly what it is—hair loss. The hair on your head falls out, and if hair on other parts of your body grows rapidly, it may also fall out (such as eyelashes or eyebrows). This is a relatively common side effect of several chemotherapy agents used to treat and manage lymphoma. Hair loss in society has become a signal that the person without hair may be a cancer patient. It can be psychologically and physically difficult to cope with hair loss because hair is associated with our self-image, health status, and other personal issues related to how we feel about our hair. Getting a wig in advance of hair loss can be helpful so that your hair style, texture, and color can be matched well for you.

Hair loss frequently starts 2½ weeks after the start of intensive chemotherapy. It is wise to keep a towel on your chair and on your pillow during that time to collect the hair that is falling out.

Some insurance companies cover the expense of a wig. Check your policy and see if your insurance company covers "skull prosthesis for side effects of cancer treatment." Costs that are not covered are tax deductible. There are programs like "Look Good, Feel Good" that most cancer centers offer to their patients. This is a special program for women, available free of charge, to show you how to wear turbans, scarves, and makeup to reduce the obvious appearance of hair loss. Ask your doctor or nurse whether they offer this program at the facility where you are getting your treatment. If the chemotherapy agents your doctor is recommending are known to cause hair loss, you can anticipate this happening between days 14 and 20 of your first chemotherapy treatment.

Some patients decide to be proactive and take charge of their hair loss themselves rather than waiting for it to happen. Getting hair cut short is a good idea. Even doing your own "buzz cut" can be therapeutic so that you determine when you lose your hair rather than waiting for the drug to do it. For women, consider having a coming out party for your head. This is a great way for friends and family to participate by bringing to you (or for children to make for you) various hats and head coverings.

INFECTION

When harmful bacteria, viruses, or fungi enter the body and the body cannot fight back to destroy these cells using the immune system, an infection brews. Lymphoma patients are at higher risk of developing an infection because the cancer along with the treatments can weaken their immune system. Symptoms that suggest infection include spiking a high fever, chills, sweating, sore throat, mouth sores, pain or burning during urination, diarrhea, shortness of breath, a productive cough, or swelling, redness, or pain around an incision or wound. With most chemotherapeutic agents, you are most at risk of infection when the white blood cell count is suppressed to its lowest point, usually between days 7 and 14 of a 14- to 21-day regimen. In some cases, this can be minimized by subcutaneous injection of a drug (Neulasta) 24 hours after chemotherapy and by preventive antibiotics during the time of risk. It is also typical for physicians to prescribe preventative drugs to avoid certain infections during therapy:

- Bactrim (prevents *Pneumocystis carnii/jiroveci* pneumonia)

- Acyclovir, Famvir, Valtrex (prevents herpes simplex and zoster)

- Diflucan (fluconazole) (prevents fungal infections)

To help reduce risk of infection, stay away from young children who may be carriers of flu viruses, colds, and other respiratory illnesses. Though they can look relatively healthy, young children may be harboring germs. This doesn't mean you need to abandon seeing your children or grandchildren. It does mean you should evaluate the child for any symptoms (runny nose, fever, cough) that would signal to you that this isn't a good day to have the child sitting on your lap. Family members who live with you or who you frequently see should get flu vaccinations to help reduce the risk of unknowingly bringing viruses your way. Frequent hand-washing by family members can help decrease the spread of infection.

If you identify any signs that you may be getting an infection (fever, cold, etc.), notify your doctor for possible examination, prescriptions, or hospitalization. During the period of greatest risk (days 7–14 after chemotherapy), any fever should be handled immediately. At a minimum, a broad-spectrum antibiotic should be taken and your physicians should be notified. Patients may require emergent evaluation and possible hospitalization. Ignoring a fever or delaying physician notification (until the morning or after the weekend) could have fatal consequences

FATIGUE

Feeling exhausted or extremely tired is probably the most common side effect patients report. This can happen as a side effect of chemotherapy and/or radiation therapy. Fatigue can also be triggered by anemia (see the next section). If you are experiencing specific problems related to fatigue, such as difficulty sleeping, make your doctor aware so that he or she can prescribe a sleep aid. Also ask about how to better cope with your emotional distress, which can increase fatigue. Conserving your energy is important so you can spend your time doing things that are important to you. Make a list of the activities and chores you are trying to accomplish (food shopping, work, house cleaning, etc.) and see about recruiting help of family and friends to assist you. You may also notice that your energy is better during certain times of the day.

ANEMIA

Anemia is a common problem for many dealing with cancer. It is especially an issue for those undergoing chemotherapy. By definition, anemia is an abnormally low level of red blood cells. These cells contain hemoglobin (an iron protein) that provides oxygen to all parts of the body. If red blood cell levels are low, parts of the body may not receive all the needed oxygen to work and function well. In general, people with anemia commonly report feeling tired or short of breath, especially on exertion. The fatigue that is associated with anemia can seriously affect quality of life for some patients and make it difficult for them to cope at times.

Medications such as Procrit (epoetin alfa) and Epogen (epoetin alfa) or Aranesp (darbepoetin) may be recommended to stimulate your bone marrow to make more red blood cells, raising your blood cell count and increasing your energy level. Such a medication is given by injection under the skin using a very small, thin needle. The doses vary, and it is common to be given one of these medications once a week or once every several weeks depending on the medication and the response of your blood counts. You might be advised to also take an iron supplement orally or intravenously while getting these injections. Alternatively, blood transfusions may be required when the anemia becomes too severe or if more rapid improvements are necessary.

CARDIAC CHANGES

Adriamycin is a chemotherapy agent that can cause future heart problems. To help evaluate if it is safe and appropriate to give these medications, a special heart scan using a MUGA (multiple-gated acquisition) scan or an echocardiogram is done before beginning therapy. Congestive heart failure, a weakness of the heart muscle, can occur but is not common. Usually, these tests are not repeated after therapy unless suggestive symptoms occur such as shortness of breath, loss of stamina, chest pain, or rapid irregular heart beats.

MOUTH SORES

Also known as mucositis, this is an inflammation of the inside of the mouth and throat and can result in painful ulcers. Certain medications like steroids may increase the risk of developing an infection in your mouth. Keep your mouth clean and moist to prevent infection. Brush your teeth with a soft-bristled toothbrush after each meal and rinse regularly. Avoid commercial mouthwashes that contain alcohol because they can irritate the mouth. If you wear dentures that are not fitting properly, you will be more likely to get sores in your mouth from rubbing and irritation. This can be a particular problem if you have experienced or are experiencing weight loss because your gums may shrink, changing the fit of your dentures. See your dentist for evaluation of this issue. If you have dental needs that have not been taken care of before starting chemotherapy, ask your oncologist and dentist to talk on the phone and discuss what strategy to use to reduce risk of infection and mouth sores while receiving your treatments.

NEUROLOGICAL PROBLEMS

Peripheral neuropathy is a term you might hear about as a possible side effect of some chemotherapy drugs. This term describes damage to peripheral nerves. There are three types of peripheral nerves: sensory, motor, and autonomic. Sensory nerves allow us to feel temperature, pain, vibration, and touch. Motor nerves are responsible for voluntary movement and basically allow us to walk and open doors, for example. Autonomic nerves control involuntary or automatic functions such as breathing, digestion of food, and bowel and bladder activities. When there is damage to the peripheral nerves, the symptoms depend on the type of peripheral nerves affected. Though chemotherapy drugs can affect any of the peripheral nerves, the most common ones affected are the sensory nerves, causing numbness and tingling in the hands and feet. For patients who already have peripheral neuropathy from other causes (diabetes, for example) the chemotherapy can sometimes make it worse. Symptoms of peripheral neuropathy include:

- Numbness and tingling (which may feel like pins and needles in your hands and/or feet)
- Burning pain in hands and feet
- Difficulty writing or buttoning a shirt
- Difficulty holding a cup or glass
- Constipation
- Decreased sensation of hot or cold
- Muscle weakness
- Decreased hearing or ringing in the ears (known as tinnitus)

If you develop any of these symptoms it is important to tell your doctor right away. Describe the symptoms you are experiencing. If you already have any of these symptoms before starting chemotherapy, make your doctor aware of that too. Your doctor may decide to prescribe medication to reduce these symptoms. The medicines most commonly used are drugs given to neurology patients for treatment of seizures and depression and may include one or several of the following: Neurontin (gabapentin), Tegretol (carbamazepine), Elavil (amitriptyline), and Lyrica (pregabalin). Some additional measures to take at home include paying close attention to your walking and removing all scatter rugs in your house. Keep your home well lit so you can see where you are walking. If you are still driving a car, be sure you can actually feel the foot pedals. If temperatures are hard to decipher, then ask for help in checking the temperature of the bathtub as well as hot beverages you are drinking. One trick is to test the temperature of water using your elbow.

LOSS OF OVARIAN OR TESTICULAR FUNCTION AND SEXUAL DYSFUNCTION

Premenopausal women who are undergoing chemotherapy may lose ovarian function and enter menopause. This is caused by a loss of estrogen and other hormones. Women under age 30 are much less likely to enter menopause, but the risk is still based on the intensity of planned chemotherapy. Some regimens, such as ABVD (Adriamycin, bleomycin, vinblastine, dacarbazine for HL), R-CVP (Rituxan, Cytoxan, Oncovin, prednisone), or FCR (fludarabine, Cytoxan, Rituxan) are unlikely to induce menopause. Other regimens, such as R-CHOP (Rituxan, Cytoxan, Adriamycin, Oncovin, prednisone), R-ICE (Rituxan, Ifex, carboplatin, etoposide), or an autologous stem cell transplantation are more likely to induce menopause. Women at high risk of lost fertility can consider banking their eggs in some cases (when the disease is not overly aggressive and widespread, mandating emergent treatment). Speak with your doctor or gynecologist for more information on egg banking.

Menopausal symptoms can range from hot flashes, night sweats, vaginal dryness, pain during intercourse, difficulty with bladder control, insomnia, and depression. Some patients take various forms of complementary therapies to try to reduce symptoms. These include vitamins, soy products, black cohosh, and other preparations. Presently, there are no studies to give us definitive answers about the use of these supplements. It is worth talking to your doctor, however, about his or her thoughts regarding your trying various supplements if you wish to consider taking any. Some patients find that taking a medication like Effexor (venlafaxine) can help reduce hot flashes. Other medications in the same drug category as this one, antidepressants, may be recommended instead to help reduce hot flashes. Wearing cotton clothing in layers that can be peeled off as needed also can be a useful measure on your part. There are various vaginal lubricants that can be used for vaginal dryness and pain during intercourse. These include Replens, Astroglide, or K-Y Jelly. Avoid using petroleum-based products because this can increase risk of vaginal infections. Avoid spicy foods, smoking, alcohol, caffeine, hot showers, and hot weather, all of which can trigger hot flashes.

Men receiving a regimen with high risk of sterility can consider sperm banking before therapy. This is usually feasible except in the most aggressive presentations of lymphoma. Sexual function for men is usually preserved, but decreased libido is common. Treatment with androgens to boost libido is an option but also carries other risks (such as higher rates of prostate cancer) in older men.

The percentage of men and women dealing with lymphoma who experience problems with continuing sexual activity is not clearly known. Even for the general population, almost half of men and women have reported problems with sexual activity for a myriad of reasons. Some patients find it very difficult to comfortably discuss this issue with their doctor, though it may be very important to their quality of life. Side effects from treatment may result in lowering of libido. Sometimes hair loss, weight gain, or fatigue cause you to simply not feel well enough to try or confident enough to engage in sexual activity. Physical intimacy is one aspect of a loving relationship. It gives us personal pleasure and creates a feeling of closeness to our partner. Sexual intercourse is just one way of being physically intimate. Cuddling, hugging, touching, rubbing, and holding hands are all pleasurable ways of showing one another affection. Talk with your partner about your concerns and feelings. This will help both of you to know how to help one another.

Experiment with different positions too, finding that one may be more comfortable than another when having sex. Vaginal lubricants (discussed earlier) can help with vaginal dryness. Some women who have not had success with vaginal lubricants have tried egg whites for lubrication. (Be sure to wash thoroughly after intercourse. Do not use douche solutions, however.) If lack of energy impairs sexual activity, plan ahead for intimacy by identifying when you are feeling higher levels of energy during certain times of the day or week. Vaginal discharge, burning, or itching may be signs of a vaginal infection. See your gynecologist if you develop these symptoms so they can be properly treated.

COGNITIVE DYSFUNCTION

Some refer to this as "chemo brain." People dealing with cancer who are getting chemotherapy as part of their treatment can have trouble remembering names, places, and events or have trouble with concentration or arithmetic. This is currently an area of scientific study to better understand what is causing it and how to counteract it. If you find that these symptoms are pretty severe and impact your ability to function well, ask your family to assist you with balancing your checkbook. Make a list of things you need to do and mark each item off as you do it. Keep your keys in the same place so they are easier to find. Most importantly, get your family members to assist you with medication management. A pill box that has the times of day to take your medications is a good idea rather than relying on your memory. After chemotherapy is completed, in time these symptoms usually subside. It's of importance to note that some patients who have not had chemotherapy report having these symptoms too. Researchers have therefore questioned whether part of the problem with remembering and with concentration could be related to stress, often referred to as posttraumatic syndrome. Remember, you are going to war with your lymphoma, so it makes sense to some degree that just like a soldier returning from the battlefield, things can feel foggy for a bit.

LYMPHEDEMA

This is an abnormal collection of lymph fluid in the arms or legs. Lymphatic fluid is in our bodies to try to fight infection and cancer. When lymph nodes in relatively large numbers have been surgically removed or radiated, however, the pathway for lymphatic drainage can become disrupted and fluid that is sent down the arm, for example, may have trouble returning back up the arm. This results in the limb swelling and staying that way. Infection, trauma to the arm, or other factors may trigger the lymphedema. Lymphedema can cause discomfort, pain, and limit the use of your limb due to swelling. The incidence of lymphedema is lower in the last 15 years because of improvements in surgical and radiation therapy techniques. If you develop lymphedema, you may experience heaviness, throbbing pain, soreness, or a feeling of tightness in your arm or leg. The following prevention steps help reduce the risk of developing lymphedema:

- Perform gentle strengthening and stretching exercises to keep the affected limb working normally.

- Avoid lifting or moving heavy objects with the affected arm after surgery.

- Keep skin clean and moisturized, avoid cuts or cracks in the skin, and avoid insect bites whenever possible.

- Avoid getting any needle sticks in the affected arm— try to avoid IVs, vaccinations, or blood draws from the arm where lymph nodes were surgically removed and/or radiated.

- Avoid getting blood pressures taken in the affected arm.

- Report signs of infection to your doctor right away. If you do get a cut or injury to this arm, wash the cut immediately and apply over-the-counter antibiotic ointment right away.

- Report any changes you notice to the affected arm, such as swelling or feeling of heaviness.

If you develop lymphedema, several treatments may be helpful. These treatments include elevation of the limb, use of special compression garments (known as compression sleeves), massage by a rehabilitation therapist who specializes in lymphedema management, compression bandaging, and a pressure pump. For more information about lymphedema, contact the National Lymphedema Network at 800-541-3259 or visit their Web site at http://www.lymphnet.org.

GASTROINTESTINAL PROBLEMS

Chemotherapy can cause either diarrhea or constipation. More than three liquid stools per day can usually be handled with loperamide orally—two to start and one after each liquid stool up to eight or nine times a day (check this limit with your doctor). Careful attention to replacing fluid and salt should prevent dehydration. Severe constipation is a feared complication of the vinca class of chemotherapy (especially vincristine), particularly in older patients. Prevention is easier than fixing the problem, and stool softeners and stimulants are recommended to keep stool soft and semisolid at the time of chemotherapy administration.

Agents include Colace (docusate sodium) and Senokot (senna) for prevention (both given once or twice a day) and MiraLax (polyethylene glycol 3350) or sorbitol for treatment.

LUNG PROBLEMS

Lung damage can occur with the use of bleomycin, which is one of the primary drugs used for Hodgkin's lymphoma. To avoid this complication, patients who receive this chemotherapy agent should get pulmonary function tests, including a single-breath diffusing capacity, and should have these parameters followed for major decrements after every two to four doses (more frequently for those at higher risk, such as smokers or ex-smokers and the elderly).

TUMOR LYSIS SYNDROME

Aggressive lymphomas and some bulky low-grade lymphomas might melt too rapidly with therapy, causing a toxic buildup of waste products, particularly uric acid, which can damage the kidneys. Before starting systemic treatment (with Rituxan, chemotherapy, or prednisone), almost all patients with lymphoma are given oral allopurinol to prevent this uric acid excess. High-risk patients should be monitored for tumor lysis syndrome at 24–48 hours, and an intravenous medication that degrades uric acid, Elitek (rasburicase), is also available.

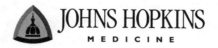

CHAPTER 5

STRAIGHT TALK—
COMMUNICATION WITH FAMILY, FRIENDS, AND COWORKERS

The feelings of shock, concern, and confusion you felt when you were diagnosed with lymphoma will also be experienced by friends and loved ones when they hear the news. Whom you will tell and when you will tell them will be different depending on their relationship to you and how they will be impacted by your news. Family members, your boss, close friends, or others who live with you will be aware that you are experiencing great stress. Your treatment is likely to change their routines as well as your own and have an emotional impact on them.

TALKING WITH CHILDREN

How and when to tell a child his or her parent has cancer is a difficult decision, no matter what the age of the child. Undoubtedly, your children will realize that something difficult is going on. It is best to be honest with your children, because they are likely to overhear conversations, even if you do not talk to them directly. Keeping the truth from your children will likely make them more scared than comforted. Depending on your family, it may make sense for either or both parents to talk with the children. Explain to them in clear terms what treatment will do to get rid of the cancer. Many parents choose to wait to tell their children until after they've seen the doctors and know the treatment plans. It is important to remember that some treatments may alter your physical appearance, and it is important to ready your children or grandchildren for that possibility. For example, if the child has never seen you without a beard, it is a good idea to shave the beard before chemotherapy so they can get used to one change at a time.

Depending on the age and maturity level of the child and on how well they are reacting to your diagnosis, it may be worth considering attending a support group for patients with lymphoma before your treatment. In addition, many major cancer centers offer educational programs for children to introduce them to the hospital and treatments to help reduce their fears and anxieties regarding the unknown. If your child has many questions about your treatment, attending such a program may help to reduce their fears and uncertainty. This is especially useful if you are scheduled for a peripheral stem cell transplantation or another intensive therapy requiring frequent visits or stays in the hospital.

TALKING WITH YOUNG CHILDREN

Toddlers and preschoolers are very dependent on their parents and as a result are quick to notice stress or tension in the home. Don't assume that their age prevents them from feeling your stress. Though children of this age won't understand what cancer is, you can let them know you are very sick and that the doctors are working very hard to make you better. Your young child may be worried that you will go away like other relatives who have passed on. Though you may not be able to assure them this will not happen to you, acknowledging their fears may be critical to their well-being. They may also feel as though something they did caused you to be ill. It is important to reassure the child that your illness is not their fault. It is a good idea to tell your child that sometimes you will feel sad or tired and that this is also not their fault. Let them know it is okay for them to be sad and that they can talk to you or your spouse any time they are feeling sad. Try to maintain family routines as much as possible.

TALKING WITH OLDER CHILDREN AND TEENS

If your children are older, they may be anxious or even angry about how this will impact them. Teens often view the world as revolving around them, and they may feel resentful about how changes in routine will impact them. These natural teen responses can be magnified by their fear of losing a parent. Because every child is different, it is important to know where your child is coming from mentally and emotionally. Keeping communication lines open is critical, particularly for children in this age group. You will have to decide who will tell the kids and when, but also how much detail you want to share with them and at what intervals. Their knowledge of lymphoma or cancer in general may be to associate it with death. Ask your child what they know about cancer and then provide them with details at their level. Reassure them honestly about your treatment and prognosis.

Teens may be particularly resentful when asked to help out around the house. There is some evidence that teens are unable to psychologically cope with the responsibility of filling a parent's role during such times of upheaval. The teen may then feel guilty about their feelings of resentment, further compounding an unfortunate situation. Find ways for the older child to contribute to the family while maintaining typical roles and boundaries as much as possible. Explain to them that you may need extra help around the house for a while, but also take steps to show balance between family responsibilities and normal teenage lifestyles. Discuss how the family will work to balance responsibilities.

TELLING OTHER FAMILY MEMBERS

Telling other family members can also be difficult. Parents in particular are used to making everything better for their children and may want to try to control the situation for you. They may be frustrated when they can't guide or control your treatment and recovery. They will need to be given constructive ways to help because no matter what, they will want to help you—even if you feel you don't need it. Parents of a patient can fill an important role in the home if there are children to care for.

Other family members will also have unique relationships that need to be considered. Siblings may feel great grief and concern for your well-being. Having them assist with information gathering can help engage them in your treatment and empower them with information that will help both of you. Family can also be critical for providing and coordinating assistance during your treatment. Remember that every offer for assistance is genuine and be ready to accept help. Keep your family members informed of how you are doing as treatment progresses. Remember, this is a disease that affects the entire family. The feelings of fear and apprehension you have are shared by many.

WHAT TO TELL YOUR BOSS AND COWORKERS

Whether or not to inform coworkers about your illness is a very personal decision. There are advantages to letting key people know because you will more than likely require some time off for treatment. You may choose to tell only your boss and your closest friends, or you may decide to be very public about your situation.

It is common to be concerned about maintaining your job after treatment. Fortunately, the Americans with Disabilities Act (ADA) provides some job protection. You and your boss should be able to work on a schedule to meet your medical needs as well as the needs of your employer. You are not actually required to tell your boss you have cancer. It is fine to explain that you are under doctor's care that will require you to miss time from work. Most individuals tell their boss they have been diagnosed with cancer and will be undergoing whatever treatments have been recommended. You are not obligated to provide information about your prognosis.

As with friends and family, deciding what to tell coworkers can be difficult. Many people choose to inform coworkers in vague terms rather than providing full details of their treatment plan. Again, this is your personal business and whatever feels right in your situation is the best answer. As with family, offers of assistance from friends and coworkers are typically genuine, and it is beneficial for you as well as those offering help to involve them as needed.

During and after treatment the need to update people on your situation can be a job in and of itself. You may want to assign someone to be the "information center" to provide all announcements about how you are doing, what treatment you are having, pathology results, and so on. There are also a number of online resources for posting such information such as http://www.caringbridge.com, a free, personalized Web site that keeps friends and family informed during difficult times. The Web site includes a patient care journal to update family and friends and a photo gallery and guest book where visitors can post messages of support and encouragement. E-mail is another good way to make sure that everyone is receiving the same information at the same time and in the same manner. A family member or friends can gather important e-mail addresses and send out broadcast e-mails to everyone at once. You will find such options to be a great time saver to help reduce the burden on you and ensure consistency in the information provided. It also helps prevent hurt feelings and discontent if one person finds out you called someone else first.

HOW TO RECRUIT SUPPORT FROM FAMILY AND FRIENDS

People will undoubtedly ask what they can do to help you. It may be beneficial to identify a coordinator early on who can delegate tasks to friends and family who want to help. Among the many things people can do are drive you to appointments, drive your children to school and events, run errands, make meals for your freezer, baby-sit, help with the housework, or add you to prayer lists at your house of worship. Remember that these people want to do something to help and would not offer if they did not sincerely want to provide assistance. One day, perhaps you will be able to reciprocate and help them in a crisis as well.

On the other hand, some friends may avoid calling you after they hear the news. It isn't that they don't care; it's more likely they don't know what to say. Let them know that even though the diagnosis is upsetting to hear, you need their support. Remember that support from others is an important part of your treatment plan for you and your family.

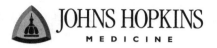

CHAPTER 6

MAINTAINING BALANCE— WORK AND LIFE DURING TREATMENT

HOW TO PLAN CARE AND MINIMIZE DISRUPTIONS IN YOUR LIFE

Modern life is hectic, requiring coordination between career, family, and personal time. Lymphoma treatment is going to alter roles, play havoc with schedules, and create additional stress for you, your family members, and your friends helping during this time. It is inevitable but manageable. Patients with children especially may experience a variety of role changes. A different partner may be putting young children to bed because the other parent doesn't feel well at night. Older children may be asked to help with meal preparation or laundry. It's important for you and your family to talk about your schedules and how treatment needs will impact everyone. The family should design a new schedule to best meet your needs and those of your loved ones—with as little change as possible. This is also the time to ask for and accept help from other family members, neighbors, and friends. After all, one day they may need your help in a very similar way.

Try to maintain your children's routines as much as possible. Change creates stress no matter what your age. Even an infant who is fed an hour later than usual expresses opinions about his or her altered schedule. Let your children know in advance of changes in their routine. Keep children informed about what is happening related to treatment. Encourage them to help and play an active role in the treatment, too. Have younger children (ages 6–12) go with you to the hospital when you get one of your chemotherapy treatments to better understand what is happening. Ask them how they picture the chemotherapy traveling through your veins destroying any bad cells that might be lingering somewhere. Have them draw pictures to cheer you up. They can open the get-well cards you receive in the mail. Explain why you don't feel well and the importance of playing quietly on certain days after treatment. Let young children know they can't catch lymphoma and also aren't in any way the cause of it.

If you are scheduled to have chemotherapy and/or immunotherapy, make a chart of when your treatments will occur. See about having chemotherapy appointments toward the end of the week so you can have the weekend to rest up (when hopefully there will be additional help around the house available to you). Decide if you want someone to go with you for chemotherapy treatments. You will be in the chemotherapy infusion center for several hours, so plan accordingly. The day needs to be as laid back as possible for you. Depending on who is available to help and what your schedules are, you may decide the chemotherapy days are when you order pizza for the kids' dinner or when you pull the casserole your neighbor made out of the freezer.

Hair loss can occur between days 16 and 30 after the first cycle of intensive chemotherapy, although many regimens and immunotherapy alone do not result in hair loss. Especially for women at risk for losing hair, if you want to be proactive, consider cutting your hair short or even doing your own buzz cut before your hair falls out on its own. A "coming out" party for your hair is fun for kids to do for you. Friends and family bring you various head coverings—turbans, hats, and so on. Your kids can make you some funny ones for wearing in the privacy of your own home.

For radiation, consider scheduling it at either the very beginning of the day or end of the day rather than in the middle. Because this is a daily treatment, you want it to disrupt your daily routine as little possible. Most radiation facilities have patients in and out in less than 30 minutes. You spend more time getting your clothes on and off than you do actually getting your treatment.

CONTINUING WORK

Most people continue to work while receiving their treatment, but this certainly depends on the intensity of the regimen. Time missed from work is usually minimal, if planned out relatively well. It actually is to your advantage to continue to work because stopping work can be an additional stress for you. You need to continue to feel productive, to be surrounded by supportive coworkers, and to be distracted from thinking about your lymphoma. Sit down with your boss and plan out a schedule that works for both of you. There may be some days you only work half a day because you are getting chemotherapy in the afternoon and then taking off the following day. During radiation you may be coming in an hour later to work or leaving 30 minutes early to get to your daily radiation appointment. Bosses know the importance of being flexible, and you are protected to some degree by the Family Medical Leave Act. If you work around small children, especially toddler age, this may be problematic during chemotherapy because your risk of getting an infection is increased during this time.

WHEN YOU MIGHT EXPECT NOT TO FEEL WELL

Usually, if you are going to have nausea, it will be 16–48 hours after the infusion of the chemotherapy drugs has been completed. How you tolerate the first chemotherapy sets the stage for how the others using the same medicines will go. Request antinausea medicines in advance, so you can also head off nausea symptoms before their occurrence.

For the time period you will be receiving radiation, if it is part of your treatment plan, anticipate feeling fine until about the last 2 weeks or so of radiation. At this point you may notice increased fatigue. This is because radiation is cumulative. Give yourself extra time to rest at night and even take a cat nap in the middle of the day if possible.

INFECTION PREVENTION

On certain days your white blood cells will go down in response to having received chemotherapy. These are days you are more vulnerable to getting a cold, flu, or other form of infection. You want to avoid being in the presence of youngsters because they can be sick but may not show any obvious symptoms. Wearing a mask is beneficial if you cannot avoid being around them in a closed environment.

Eating a balanced diet, rich in fruits and vegetables, helps to improve your immune system. Washing your hands frequently is smart. When feasible, getting a flu shot or other immunizations before you start chemotherapy is advisable. Any dental work that needs to be done should happen before you start chemotherapy to prevent a problem related to tooth infections later. Chemotherapy doesn't cause dental problems but may aggravate preexisting ones due to the immune system being taxed and unable to fight infection as well as it did before. If you need to travel by air while undergoing chemotherapy, wear a mask to reduce risk of exposure. If it is winter, be sure to have yourself bundled up when outdoors. Your mission is to be healthy during your chemotherapy treatments and to reduce risk of exposure to infection as much as possible. The nurse working with you during your chemotherapy treatments can mark on your chart the days you will be particularly vulnerable to infection. Your blood will be periodically drawn to assess how your body's immune system is responding to the treatments and whether any medicines to boost your white blood cells need to be given.

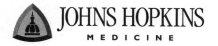

CHAPTER 7

Surviving Lymphoma— Re-engaging in Mind and Body Health After Treatment

SURVIVORSHIP

When do you consider yourself to be a survivor? The most common definition is actually the moment you are diagnosed and have chosen to embark on treatment or careful monitoring. Some patients, especially those with aggressive lymphoma or with symptomatic indolent lymphoma, consider themselves survivors when they have attained a complete remission after treatment is over. You are not alone. There are over a million lymphoma patients who are cured or living with their disease with a great quality of life.

When you finish your treatment, rather than feeling like celebrating you may feel like you fell off a cliff. You've been so focused on actively fighting this disease that when it's time to stop, you feel a sense of disappointment. You may be fearful that you haven't done enough, or that there isn't additional treatment to continue to take as a means of preventing recurrence. Some require additional maintenance treatments, whereas others are considered free of disease without need for further therapy. Fear of recurrence remains the biggest issue that survivors have to deal with today. It can be hard to learn to trust your body again. Staying informed about the latest published research on lymphoma is helpful and empowering. It is also wise to take measures to help regain your emotional balance. Some cancer support groups, such as the American Cancer Society, offer special survivor retreats for this purpose.

COUNSELING

If your doctor or nurse recommends that you consider seeing a counselor, don't feel like you failed at getting yourself back on track. Many individuals benefit from seeing a therapist to help them re-engage in their physical and emotional lives. Sometimes patients just need a professional sounding board to hear their hidden thoughts and fears and help them gain perspective about what is important. To regain control over your life, you may require assistance from others who are professionally trained in this area. Diagnosis and treatment of lymphoma is a life-altering experience that does not come with an operator's manual. It is also helpful to talk with other survivors to realize that what you are experiencing is the norm and not the exception.

MANAGING LONG-TERM SIDE EFFECTS OF TREATMENT

Often, after treatment ends the side effects associated with it do not. You may be dealing with residual side effects of bone or joint pain, numbness and tingling of the fingers and toes, difficulty concentrating, fatigue, hot flashes, night sweats, or other unpleasantness. Give your body time to heal and adjust. Some side effects like fatigue can linger for a year or longer. Premenopausal women may experience menopausal symptoms due to therapy. Don't expect to feel normal the week treatments end. There is a period of psychological and physical adjustment, similar to a woman becoming pregnant and 9 months later giving birth. Your body needs time. Allow it this time. (See Chapter 4 for management of side effects.)

LIVING A HEALTHIER LIFESTYLE

Taking charge of your health and psychological well-being should now be your priority. In this section we discuss some helpful ways to accomplish this and to feel good about doing it.

NUTRITION

If you eat healthier and watch your weight, you may help to reduce your risk of other illnesses that could interfere with future treatment. Although there is no evidence to date that any specific diet prevents recurrence or encourages responses to therapy or to observation, avoiding high-fat foods is a good policy to prevent weight gain and to protect your heart. This doesn't mean giving up chocolate ice cream sundaes for the rest of your life. Eat smart. Save high-fat and high-calorie foods for special times and rewards.

If you are currently overweight, consider joining a group to help you reduce weight gradually. Avoid diet pills and fad diets. Changing eating habits and making it part of your lifestyle is the way to take the weight off and keep it off. It needs to be an overall program and not something temporary.

People usually have better success at losing weight when they partner with someone else who shares the same goal.

EXERCISE

This is another way to help control your weight and regain your strength. This doesn't mean you need to become a marathon runner and press 400 pounds at the gym. It does mean finding an exercise program that works for you, that you can commit to, and that makes you feel good. If you enjoy the exercise program, if it is in an environment that makes you feel comfortable, if you feel better after you do it, and if it is something you are able to stick with, then it's a winner for you. Power walking is one option to consider. Walking or working out three times a week for an hour will suffice. Again, exercising with a friend usually makes it more enjoyable and helps you to persevere because you have a buddy rooting you on.

STRESS

Emotional turmoil affects our immune system and our immune system needs to be in good shape to fight the immune-related cancer cells and prevent cancer cells from growing. You will be expected to resume your chaotic life, including family responsibilities and work duties. Having lymphoma can teach us that we really don't have to sweat the small stuff. Many individuals realize that they had misplaced priorities and unnecessary anxieties over less critical issues. Making time for you is important, including after treatment is completed. Put things into perspective before reacting to them. Is it really a crisis that your mother-in-law is moving in for a month? You've been through much bigger and more significant stuff. Learn deep-breathing techniques, take a yoga class, or learn other forms of relaxation therapy that can be helpful to you in reducing stress and keeping life in perspective.

AVOID SMOKE AND ALCOHOL

This includes secondary smoke. If you have friends who smoke, remind them that if they care about you they will take their cigarettes outside. If they refuse and still smoke around you, then they aren't your friends. Limit your alcohol intake to only one or two drinks a day.

SETTING NEW GOALS

You may have just completed treatment that was life altering. You have perhaps stared death in the face and survived what you thought wasn't possible to overcome. Perhaps you have a very slow-growing lymphoma and you are facing decades of future observation or therapy. This is an ideal time to step back and reassess your life, looking at how you want to leave your mark on this earth, now realizing you are going to be around to make that mark. It's your call. It's your life. Consider setting both short-term and long-term goals. Some goals may be directed at living a healthier lifestyle; others may be focused on how you want to make a difference for others who come after you and are diagnosed with lymphoma. You are connected to an extraordinary group of lymphoma survivors who share common thoughts, dreams, and fears. Band together to make a difference or strike out on your own. When you consider how you want to spend the rest of your life, what you thought was important before may have little meaning now. This can be quite confusing to those around you who were expecting things to return to "normal." You need to find your "new normal" and let your family and friends know you are working hard to accomplish this. This experience has changed you, hopefully for the better, in that life will be considered more precious and valued than it was before. You have gotten in touch with your mortality, no doubt about it. Communicate your thoughts with your family and friends. Consider keeping a journal to record your ideas.

SEEING THE WORLD THROUGH DIFFERENT EYES

It can be hard for people you spend time with—family, friends, and coworkers—to realize you aren't the same person you were before your diagnosis. Hopefully you are different in all the right ways, now mindful of how precious life is and how your health is your most precious possession. Never take anything for granted. Value your relationships perhaps differently from what you did before. Consider getting involved as a volunteer. One of the best ways to move forward with your experience with lymphoma is to help those who are diagnosed after you. By helping someone else, you help yourself psychologically; consider volunteering near where you received your treatments or volunteer for a cancer organization that has a chapter in your area. This is very rewarding and a great way to give back; it can help others as well as yourself. Educate others and help promote lymphoma research.

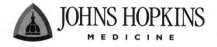

CHAPTER 8

MANAGING RISK—
WHAT IF MY LYMPHOMA
COMES BACK?

Risk of progression or recurrence remains the most feared issue for individuals when they have finished their treatment. Learning what to look for, when, how, and for how long is helpful. Putting risk of progression or recurrence into perspective is extremely important to your psychological well-being. For example, constantly pressing areas of current or prior lymph node involvement can irritate and swell even normal lymph nodes, causing needless pain and inflammation, as well as unnecessary fear of possible recurrence. A simple and effective rule is to allow yourself one gentle exploration per day at most. The truth is that any meaningful progression or recurrence will become obvious in a matter of days or weeks even without active surveillance. More importantly, any such delay in detection will not worsen your prognosis. You will respond just as well with retreatment when the delay is only a matter of days or weeks.

MONITORING FOR PROGRESSION OR RECURRENCE

Risk of progression or recurrence depends on the type of lymphoma (indolent or aggressive), the stage at presentation, and any history of prior treatment and their results. Special prognostic scales (such as the International Prognostic Index or specific versions) and new genetic and immunological factors can also help to define the risk of progression or recurrence. This risk, in turn, translates into the proper schedule for follow-up and testing.

DIFFERENT RISK SCENARIOS

As examples, we present various scenarios you may be able to match with your own. However, the combination of factors is too complex to provide a "one size fits all" set of scenarios. Your physician and healthcare team can best advise you about a reasonable schedule that is individualized for your specific parameters.

AGGRESSIVE LYMPHOMA (INCLUDING HODGKIN'S LYMPHOMA): GOOD RISK BASED ON PROGNOSTIC FACTORS, IN REMISSION AFTER CURATIVE THERAPY

You are most likely cured, but your highest risk of recurrence is in the first 2 years (80% of cases), and retreatment can still be curative. For this reason follow-up is frequent (every 3–4 months for the first 2 years) with CTs or MRIs every 6 months for 2 years and usually less frequently after that until 5 years after treatment. Visits usually include physical examination and routine blood tests (complete blood count, comprehensive metabolic panel, and any tumor markers such as lactate dehydrogenase, sedimentation rate, or associated antibody elevations, for example). There is very little evidence that this active monitoring results in any benefits; in fact, studies show that 80% of patients who recur present with symptoms in between the scans. These symptoms include recurrent fever and sweats not accounted for by a current infection, loss of weight and appetite, new lymph nodes, or unexplained pain and discomfort that is worsening over time. For the same reason, it is hard to justify the extra radiation exposure and expense of routine PETs/CTs for monitoring after therapy. These scans are reserved for higher risk situations such as recurrence of symptoms or new lymph nodes.

AGGRESSIVE LYMPHOMA (INCLUDING HODGKIN'S LYMPHOMA): POOR RISK BASED ON PROGNOSTIC FACTORS, IN REMISSION AFTER CURATIVE THERAPY

The highest risk patients may be offered further consolidation therapy (sometimes as part of a study). After that, follow-up is frequent and similar to the schedule listed for good risk patients. CAT scans or MRIs may be ordered more frequently, especially in the first year after treatment, and PET/CAT scans are used more liberally for any adverse symptoms or signs.

INDOLENT LYMPHOMA: GOOD RISK BASED ON PROGNOSTIC FACTORS, WATCHFUL WAITING

Although a cure is not the goal, you might be free of symptoms with no need for treatment for years or even decades. Many patients take this time as an opportunity to optimize their health otherwise, implementing healthy nutritional choices and an exercise program. Although there are no studies proving that healthy choices or supplemental nutrition can improve the immune system and thereby improve your prognosis, most patients and physicians embrace good health choices.

Up to 30% of patients with some indolent lymphomas (especially follicular lymphoma) may undergo spontaneous remission during a watchful waiting approach. If you happen to be taking a vitamin supplement or so-called natural herb, you may mistakenly attribute your spontaneous remission to this choice. Humans are hardwired to try to find connections in their life, and it is normal and usual to associate any good news with a directed action or choice. It is easy to imagine some people attributing their improvement to a solar eclipse that occurred during a spontaneous remission. It is easy to see how purveyors of "natural herbs" or "natural cures" could find wonderful testimonials among clients with indolent lymphoma: "It was all over her body, the doctor had no cure, and she was told that treatment would not be given. We then gave her 'Vitameatavegamin' and all the cancer areas disappeared!"

There is no standard follow-up schedule for watchful waiting. An initial schedule of visits every 4 months for physical examination and blood tests can be lengthened to every 6 months after 1–2 years. CAT scans or MRIs are not done as often as for patients with lymphoma, although new symptoms or signs would warrant a PET/CAT scan.

INDOLENT LYMPHOMA: INTERMEDIATE OR WORSE RISK DUE TO SYMPTOMS OR PROGNOSTIC FACTORS, IN REMISSION AFTER THERAPY

Most individuals with indolent lymphoma are offered maintenance treatment for several years with the immunological agent Rituxan after primary treatment with attainment of a remission. The schedule for these maintenance treatments dictates concurrent follow-up. Although many physicians order CAT scans at least yearly for the first 5 years, this decision is also based on ease of follow-up by exam or blood tests. Some indolent lymphomas first appear as a rising white blood cell count, worsening anemia (lowering red blood cell count), or enlarging lymph nodes. Again, your physician and healthcare team, in consideration of your attitude and lifestyle, can devise a program of follow-up that best meets your needs. As mentioned before, you will be the first person to detect most recurrences because symptoms and signs usually occur between visits and tests. This does not mean that you need even more visits or tests but rather that any delay in detection of recurrence is not important enough to affect prognosis. The ability to respond again and attain remission is not dependent on speed of detection.

Sometimes, more specialized or invasive testing is required on follow-up. This usually occurs as part of a clinical trial. For example, those who receive a peripheral stem cell transplantation are often monitored with periodic bone marrow testing.

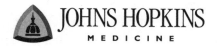

CHAPTER 9

My Lymphoma Isn't Curable— What Now?

CURE VERSUS PALLIATION: A PHILOSOPHY OF MANAGEMENT

The definition of cure can be stretched when dealing with HL and NHL. A patient with an indolent, low-grade lymphoma may live for decades without treatment, yet officially that patient is incurable in the same way as a diabetic, a hypertensive patient, or a patient with rheumatoid arthritis. On the other hand, a patient with an aggressive lymphoma might require several rounds of treatment, only to die free of disease from complications after stem cell transplantation. Who is better off?

In general, patients with indolent, low-grade lymphoma are not curable. But even this simple statement has exceptions. When indolent lymphoma is strictly localized, radiotherapy may be curative, or at least recurrences may not be evident for decades. Some younger patients with advanced-stage indolent lymphoma may be cured if they are willing to risk the mortality and side effects of stem cell transplantation from a sibling, relative, or well-matched donor. Usually, patients with indolent lymphoma over the age of 60 pursue a watchful waiting approach when possible or a very conservative approach when needed, using therapy only when required. Those patients have accepted a philosophy of palliation, which means treatment with the goal of prolonging life with quality but not aiming for a difficult cure. A goal of palliation need not be permanent. New breakthroughs and developments can inspire a physician to switch from palliative to more curative treatment. Patients with HL or aggressive lymphoma are usually curable with first-line therapy. Even relapses of these lymphomas may be curable with more aggressive measures, including stem cell transplantations. Yet the time may come for the unlucky few to turn from curative approaches to palliative approaches. Several months or years of quality life are still possible in this situation.

Oncologists and hematologists are taught that the first round of therapy buys the best quality and duration of remission, with the highest cure rates when feasible. Subsequent remissions generally are less and less durable over time, and this observation, coupled with the number of different therapies that might yet be applied and with the quality and depth of each response, can yield estimates of time left for the patient. But this is too imprecise to be any more than a general guide. A particularly effective new therapy or intensive modality, such as stem cell transplantation, might yield a particularly long remission or even a cure. Every physician can point to lymphoma patients in their practice who never followed the textbooks and have escaped dire predictions and seemingly insurmountable obstacles.

SETTING SHORT-TERM GOALS

Though it would be wonderful to make plans for 10 years from now and expect to be here to carry them out, that may not be realistic in some cases. Begin with setting short-term goals. Let's see how effectively the cancer responds to the treatment recommended. Short-term goals may be 1 year in length. Are there patients who have lived with recurrent lymphoma? Yes, and along the way new treatments extended the length and quality of life, and in some cases patients have been cured who were previously designated as incurable. No area of cancer research has seen more breakthroughs with new and exciting agents almost on a yearly basis than blood- and lymph-related malignancies. Living longer always brings hope for new and better treatments, as well as better news from the doctors. Frankly discuss with your doctor what to expect. Don't purchase cruise tickets for 3 years from now in your name that are not refundable. Be optimistic but also realistic. The goal may be for you to be here for many years, but first see how your body responds to treatment before making any assumptions. Ask the doctor how long you will be taking treatment before scans will be repeated to judge how effective the medications have been for shrinking the lymphoma.

QUALITY OF LIFE VERSUS QUANTITY OF LIFE

The mission for anyone should be to maintain a good quality of life and not just focus on how many days, weeks, or years you will be here. Quantity needs to take a back seat to quality of life. Living a long time in severe pain, unable to take care of your daily needs, and not enjoying still being alive is no way to live. A shorter length of time during which you feel pretty good and can enjoy family is far better than a longer length of time during which you are miserable. If you are experiencing a lot of pain, speak up. There are medications to control pain. The doctors and nurses may not know you are suffering if you don't tell them. Sometimes patients are frightened about reporting new symptoms like this, fearing they will hear that this means the prognosis is worse. There are situations in which giving a little bit of radiation to the spine, for example, may take back pain away completely. This can only happen by telling the doctor your symptoms and how you feel.

WHEN SHOULD I STOP TREATMENT?

This is not an easy question to ask of your doctor and not an easy question for him or her to answer. Having a candid discussion about this is very valuable. It may require meeting with your doctor one on one when family isn't accompanying you. It's sometimes easier to talk frankly without your spouse, child, or parent sitting beside you because they don't want to hear the answer to this question. There is no sense in doing treatment for treatment's sake if it isn't helping. You want your doctor to be very honest and open with you. It will be just as hard for your doctor to tell you that he or she recommends that treatment stop as it will be for you to hear those words. Physicians are trained to make patients better, to heal, to cure, to take pain away, and to reduce suffering. Having to tell someone that continuing treatment isn't going to be beneficial to accomplish any of these goals is hard but important to state if and when such a time comes. Being prepared for such a time is wise. This means asking the doctor how long he or she anticipates being able to hold the disease at bay, what drugs in what order you can anticipate being offered, and for how long, and so on. Be sure to have your affairs in order and your wishes known. There is a tendency to postpone doing this, perhaps because of denial. Everyone, whether they have lymphoma or not, should have his or her affairs in order. Life is unpredictable. Fatal accidents can happen. You are in a situation that is providing you a window into your future and what timeline it holds for you. Take advantage of this unusual knowledge and make sure that you have a will and an advanced directive, that your finances are in order, and that your wishes are clearly known to your next of kin.

HOSPICE AND PALLIATIVE CARE

When we reach end of life, there are special medical services available to help in preparing for leaving this world, dying with dignity as well as with pain in control, and having your family's emotional needs met. Hospice is such an organization that helps make this possible. A referral from your doctor is needed and commonly is arranged around the time the decision is made that treatment is no longer benefitting you. Hospice care can be provided in a hospice facility, in your home, or in a relative's home. It's your choice. Again, quality of life is paramount. Honoring your wishes and spending time as you want to spend it is the mission now. Counseling is provided to family members, and spiritual needs are addressed for everyone. This is your time with family and friends...this is your time for reflection and to gain a sense of peace.

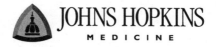

CHAPTER 10

LYMPHOMA IN OLDER ADULTS
GARY R. SHAPIRO, MD

The non-Hodgkin's lymphomas are much more common than Hodgkin's lymphoma, and their risk increases with age. NHLs are usually found in individuals older than 60, with an average age at diagnosis of around 70 years. Although the average age of patients with HL is 28, one-third of patients are older than 60. As we live longer, the number of people with all lymphomas will increase. In the next 25 years the number of people who are 65 years of age and older will double, and the largest increases in cancer incidence will occur in those older than 80 years of age.

Older adults with cancer often have other chronic health problems and may be taking multiple medications that can affect their cancer treatment plan. Prejudice, misunderstanding, and limited access to clinical trials often prevent older patients from getting the timely cancer treatment they need.

Older men and women may not have adequate screening for lymphoma, and when a cancer is found it is too often ignored or under-treated. As a result, older individuals often have more advanced stage cancer and worse outcomes than younger patients. Older patients have less chemotherapy, less radiation therapy, and their lymphoma is often left untreated.

WHY IS THERE MORE CANCER IN OLDER PEOPLE?

The organs in our body are made up of cells. Cells divide and multiply as the body needs them. Cancer develops when cells in a part of the body grow out of control. The body has a number of ways to repair damaged control mechanisms, but as we get older these do not work as well. Although our healthier lifestyles have allowed us to avoid death from infection, heart attack, and stroke, we may now live long enough for a cancer to develop. People who live longer have increased exposure to cancer-causing agents (carcinogens) in the environment (pesticides, radiation exposure, or certain viruses such as Epstein-Barr virus [see Chapter 1]). Aging decreases the body's ability to protect us from these carcinogens and to repair cells that are damaged by these and other processes.

LYMPHOMA IS DIFFERENT IN OLDER PEOPLE

The biology of lymphoma is different in older individuals than in younger people. Older patients with HL commonly present with mixed cellularity histology, B symptoms, advanced stage, and Epstein-Barr virus–positive disease (see Chapter 1). Compared with younger patients, older people with either HL or NHLs are more likely to have disease that is resistant to treatment. Indeed, age is one of the most important risk factors, and a key indicator of survival in the International Prognostic Index (see Chapter 1).

DECISION MAKING: 7 PRACTICAL STEPS

1. GET A DIAGNOSIS

No matter how "typical" the signs and symptoms, first impressions are sometimes wrong. That swollen lymph node in your neck may well be due to an infection or some other benign problem. Although enlarged lymph nodes may be a sign of lymphoma, other types of cancer often spread to lymph nodes, and their treatment and prognosis are usually quite different. Even when lymphoma is diagnosed, it is critical that you and your doctors know just what type of lymphoma you are dealing with (see Chapter 1). For example, the aggressive types of NHL (and HL) can take your life quickly but are often cured by chemotherapy. On the other hand, the indolent NHLs are usually not curable but grow so slowly that you may live symptom free for many years without the need for any anticancer treatment at all.

An accurate diagnosis helps you and your family understand what to expect and how to prepare for the future, even if you cannot get curative treatment. Knowing the diagnosis also helps your doctor treat your symptoms better. Many people find not knowing very hard and are relieved when they finally have an explanation for their symptoms. Sometimes a frail patient is obviously dying, and diagnostic studies can be an additional burden. In such cases it may be quite reasonable to focus on symptom relief (palliation) without knowing the details of the diagnosis.

2. KNOW THE CANCER'S STAGE

Although the specific type of lymphoma that you have is the most important factor in determining your prognosis and treatment options, knowing its stage is also quite important. No one can make informed decisions without it.

95

Just as there may be times when the burdens of diagnostic studies may be too great, it may also be appropriate to do without full staging in very frail, dying patients.

As it is in younger patients, stage is determined by the number and location of lymph nodes affected by lymphoma, the presence or absence of "B" symptoms (fever, sweating, weight loss), and several other factors such as the level of LDH in your blood or whether lymphoma is in your bone marrow, liver, or other organs. When doctors combine this information with information regarding your lymphoma's subtype, they can predict what impact, if any, your lymphoma is likely to have on your life expectancy and quality of life.

3. KNOW YOUR LIFE EXPECTANCY

Anticancer treatment should be considered if you are likely to live long enough to experience symptoms or premature death from lymphoma. If your life expectancy is so short that the cancer will not significantly affect it, there may be no reason to treat your cancer.

However, chronological age (how old you are) should not be the only thing that decides how your cancer should, or should not, be treated. Despite advanced age, people who are relatively well often have a life expectancy that is longer than their life expectancy with lymphoma. The average 70-year-old woman is likely to live another 16 years and the average 70-year-old man another 12 years. A similar 85-year-old can expect to live an additional 5–6 years and remain independent for most of that time. Even an unhealthy 75-year-old man or woman probably will live 5–6 more years, long enough to suffer symptoms and early death from recurrent lymphoma.

4. UNDERSTAND THE GOALS

Goals of Treatment

It is important to be clear whether the goal of treatment is cure or palliation (radiation or chemotherapy for incurable advanced or recurrent lymphoma). If the goal is palliation, you need to understand if the treatment plan will extend your life, control your symptoms, or both. How likely is it to achieve these goals, and how long will you enjoy its benefits?

When the goal of treatment is palliation, chemotherapy should never be administered without defined endpoints and timelines. It should be clear to everyone what "counts" as success, how it will be determined (for example, a symptom controlled or a smaller mass on CT), and when. You and your family should understand what your options are at each step, and how likely each is to meet your goals. If this is not clear, ask your doctor to explain it in words you understand.

Goals of the Patient

In addition to the traditional goals of tumor response, increased survival, and symptom control, older cancer patients often have goals related to quality of life. These may include physical and intellectual independence, spending quality time with your family, taking trips, staying out of the hospital, or even economic stability. At times, palliative care or hospice may meet these goals better than active anticancer treatment. In addition to the medical team, older patients often turn to family, friends, and clergy to help guide them.

5. DETERMINE IF YOU ARE FIT OR FRAIL

Deciding how to treat cancer in someone who is older requires a thorough understanding of his or her general health and social situation. Decisions about cancer treatment should never focus on age alone.

Age Is Not a Number

Your actual age (chronological age) has limited influence on how cancer will respond to therapy or its prognosis. Biological and other changes associated with aging are more reliable in estimating an individual's vigor, life expectancy, or the risk of treatment complications. These changes include malnutrition, loss of muscle mass and strength, depression, dementia, falls, social isolation, and the inability to accomplish daily activities such as dressing, bathing, eating, shopping, housekeeping, and managing one's finances or medication.

Chronic Illnesses

Older cancer patients are likely to have chronic illnesses (comorbidity) that affect their life expectancy; the more that you have, the greater the effect. This effect has very little impact on the behavior of the cancer itself, but studies do show that comorbidity has a major impact on treatment outcome and its side effects.

6. BALANCE BENEFITS AND HARMS

Fit older lymphoma patients respond to treatment similarly to their younger counterparts. However, a word of caution is in order. Until recently, few studies included older individuals, and it may not be appropriate to apply these findings to the diverse group of older cancer patients.

The side effects of cancer treatment are never less in the elderly. In addition to the standard side effects, there are significant age-related toxicities to consider. Though most of these are more a function of frailty than chronological age, even the fittest senior cannot avoid the physical effects of aging. In addition to the changes in fat and muscle that you see in the mirror, there are age-related changes in your kidney, liver, and digestive (gastrointestinal) function. These changes affect how your body absorbs and metabolizes anticancer drugs and other medicines. The average senior takes many different medicines (to control, for example, high blood pressure, high cholesterol, osteoporosis, diabetes, arthritis, etc.). This "polypharmacy" can cause undesirable side effects as the many drugs interact with each other and the anticancer medications.

7. GET INVOLVED

Healthcare providers and family members often underestimate the physical and mental abilities of older people and their willingness to face chronic and life-threatening conditions. Studies clearly show that older patients want detailed and easily understood information about potential treatments and alternatives. Patients and families may consider cancer untreatable in the aged and not understand the possibilities offered by treatment.

Although patients with dementia pose a unique challenge, they are frequently capable of participating in goal setting and simple discussions about treatment side effects and logistics. Caring family members and friends are often able to share the patient's life story so that healthcare workers can work with them to make decisions consistent with the patient's values and desires. This of course is no substitute for a well thought out and properly executed living will or healthcare proxy.

Although it is hard to face the possibility of life-threatening events at any age, it is always better to be prepared and to "put your affairs in order." In addition to estate planning and wills, it is critical that you outline your wishes regarding medical care at the end of life and make legal provisions for someone to make those decisions if you are unable to make them for yourself.

TREATING LYMPHOMA

YOU NEED A TEAM

Cancer care changes rapidly, and it is hard for the generalist to keep up to date, so referral to a specialist is essential. The needs of an older cancer patient often extend beyond the doctor's office and the traditional services provided by visiting nurses. These needs may include transportation, nutrition, and emotional, financial, physical, and spiritual support. When an older woman or man with lymphoma is the primary caregiver for a frail or ill spouse, grandchildren, or other family members, special attention is necessary to provide for their needs as well. Older cancer patients cared for in geriatric oncology programs benefit from multidisciplinary teams of oncologists, geriatricians, psychiatrists, pharmacists, physiatrists, social workers, nurses, clergy, and dietitians, all working together as a team to identify and manage the stressors that can limit effective cancer treatment.

WATCHFUL WAITING

As discussed in Chapters 1 and 3, many men and women carry a diagnosis of indolent lymphoma that probably will not threaten their life spans. This is often the situation for older individuals who have a life expectancy of less than

10 years or whose diagnostic workup suggests low-risk disease (stage I or II, few lymph nodes, normal LDH, and no anemia). Some forms of indolent NHLs are detectable but never cause symptoms, whereas others grow progressively until symptoms appear. Indolent forms of NHLs are usually not curable, but most elderly patients' symptoms can be relieved with chemotherapy (or sometimes with radiation therapy) so they can live normal or near-normal lives for many years. Nearly three-fourths of fit seniors will be alive 10 years after they are diagnosed with a low-risk, indolent NHL, and many will remain symptom free without treatment for quite a few more years. Although only one-third of patients with high-risk NHL (stage III or IV, many lymph nodes, high LDH, and anemia) will survive more than 10 years, treatment can often wait until symptoms appear.

Aggressive forms of NHL and all forms of HL are among the fastest growing forms of cancer. Symptoms usually develop in only a few weeks. If left untreated, these types of lymphomas progress to death in only a matter of several months. Unlike the indolent types of NHL, these lymphomas are very sensitive to chemotherapy and are potentially curable. Most seniors decide that the risks of chemotherapy are worth taking. Although chemotherapy for aggressive lymphomas can be tough, there is little doubt that it is the best way to control symptoms in all but the most frail man or woman with aggressive NHL and advanced-stage HL. Radiation therapy may be a good option for those with early stages of HL (see later in this chapter).

CHEMOTHERAPY

Nonfrail older cancer patients respond to chemotherapy similarly to their younger counterparts with HL or NHL. Though the side effects of cancer treatment are never less burdensome in the elderly, they can be managed by oncologists who focus on the special concerns of the elderly. With appropriate care, healthy older men and women do just as well with chemotherapy as younger individuals. Advances in supportive care (antinausea medicines and blood cell growth factors) have significantly decreased the side effects of chemotherapy and improved safety and the quality of life of older individuals with lymphoma. Nonetheless, there is risk, especially if the patient is frail.

With regard to choice of chemotherapy, healthy older patients can receive the same regimens as their younger counterparts, including those that are anthracycline-based, like CHOP for aggressive NHL or ABVD for HL (see Chapter 3). Older patients are at increased risk of developing congestive heart failure from these regimens, and those with a significant cardiac risk need frequent monitoring, including serial echocardiograms. Unfortunately, when it comes to treating aggressive lymphomas, there are no good substitutes for anthracyclines like Adriamycin. The less intensive anthracycline-free chemotherapy regimens may provide some symptom relief for those with aggressive lymphomas, but they are usually less effective than anthracycline-based regimens. They should be reserved for patients with only the most severe cardiac disease.

Managing chemotherapy-associated toxicity with appropriate supportive care is crucial in the elderly population to give them the best chance of cure and survival or to provide the best palliation. Reducing the dose of chemotherapy (or radiation therapy) based purely on chronological age may seriously affect the effectiveness of treatment.

Although Rituxan (see Chapter 3) is usually given in combination with chemotherapy, as a single agent it may be a reasonable alternative for symptom control (palliation) in those too frail to tolerate standard regimens like R-CHOP. Even frail individuals have few side effects from Rituxan. Corticosteroids (prednisone or dexamethasone) can also be used to temporarily relieve symptoms in the frail elderly who are unable to tolerate aggressive chemotherapy or for whom long-term survival is not a realistic goal. The presence of severe comorbidities, age-related frailty, or underlying severe psychosocial problems may be obstacles, even for these palliative treatment plans.

RADIATION THERAPY

As in younger patients, radiation therapy is used as an adjunct to chemotherapy in those with large masses of malignant lymph nodes or as primary treatment for early-stage NHL (see Chapter 3). It may also be an alternative for some older patients with earlier stages of HL. Its response and cure rates are almost as good as those of chemotherapy in patients with low-risk stage I and II HL. Radiation therapy also provides excellent palliation in patients with symptoms related to localized areas of indolent NHL, like pain or obstruction due to a mass of enlarged lymph nodes. It is particularly effective in treating pain, weakness, and numbness caused by lymphoma that has spread to the bone (spinal cord compression). A short course of radiation therapy often allows patients with advanced lymphoma to lower (or even eliminate) their dose of narcotic pain relievers. Although these medicines do an excellent job of controlling pain, they often cause confusion, falls, and constipation in older patients. Thus even hospice patients suffering from localized pain (or symptoms related to masses of malignant lymph nodes obstructing blood vessels, the gastrointestinal tract, or the kidney) should consider the option of palliative radiation therapy.

The fatigue that usually accompanies radiation therapy can be quite profound in the elderly, even in those who are fit. Often, the logistical details (like daily travel to the hospital for a 6-week course of treatment) are the hardest for older people. It is important that you discuss these potential problems with your family and social worker before starting radiation therapy.

TRANSPLANT

As discussed in Chapter 3, bone marrow transplantation (or stem cell transplantation) is sometimes used to treat recurrent lymphomas or those that are refractory to standard treatment. These are extremely risky procedures, even in the young and healthy. The risks increase dramatically with greater age and are usually over the top if you have any significant comorbidity. It used to be said that anyone over 50 years old should not have a transplant, but recent advances now make it possible for carefully selected fit seniors to consider these forms of aggressive therapy, especially the autologous type of transplant procedure. Although the risks of standard allogeneic transplant are usually too great for any older person, some transplant centers include the fit elderly in their "mini transplants" (nonmyeloablative stem cell transplants) research studies.

SURGERY

Surgery is not used to treat lymphoma. However, a surgeon is often called upon to remove a lymph node so that a pathologist can determine if you have a lymphoma and its specific subtype. This diagnostic biopsy is usually done as an outpatient under local anesthesia. It is a low-risk and routine procedure that is well tolerated by even those who are quite frail.

COMMON TREATMENT COMPLICATIONS
IN THE ELDERLY

Anemia (low red blood cell count) is common in the elderly, especially the frail elderly. It decreases the effectiveness of chemotherapy and often causes fatigue, falls, cognitive decline (for example, dementia, disorientation, or confusion), and heart problems. Therefore it is essential that anemia be recognized and corrected with red blood cell transfusions or the appropriate use of erythropoiesis-stimulating agents like Procrit and Epogen or Aranesp.

Myelosuppression (low white blood cell count) is also common in older patients getting chemotherapy or radiation therapy. Older patients with myelosuppression develop life-threatening infections more often than younger patients, and they may need to be treated in the hospital for many days. The liberal use of granulopoietic growth factors (Neupogen, Neulasta) decreases the risk of infection and makes it possible for older men and women to receive full doses of potentially curable chemotherapy.

Thrombocytopenia (low platelet cell count in the blood) can cause serious bleeding problems. This is especially worrisome in an older person who is prone to falling. Someone who bleeds into the brain can suffer a serious and debilitating stroke. Like anemia and myelosuppression, thrombocytopenia is a side effect of many chemotherapy medicines (especially carboplatin) and radiation therapy. It can usually be successfully managed by checking blood counts frequently and transfusing platelets when appropriate.

Mucositis (mouth sores) and diarrhea can cause severe dehydration in older patients who often are already dehydrated due to inadequate fluid intake and diuretics ("water pills" for high blood pressure or heart failure). Careful monitoring and the liberal use of antidiarrheal agents (Imodium) and oral and intravenous fluids are essential components of the management of older cancer patients.

Kidney function declines as we age. Some of the medicines that older patients take to treat both their cancer (for example, Platinol AQ (cisplatin), Paraplatin (carboplatin), zoledronic acid, nonsteroidal anti-inflammatory drugs) and noncancer-related problems might make this worse. The dehydration that often accompanies cancer and its treatment can put additional stress on the kidneys. Fortunately, it is often possible to minimize these effects by carefully selecting and dosing appropriate drugs, managing "polypharmacy," and preventing dehydration.

Neurotoxicity and cognitive effects ("chemo brain") can be profoundly debilitating in patients who are already cognitively impaired (demented, disoriented, confused, etc.). Elderly patients with a history of falling, hearing loss, or peripheral neuropathy (nerve damage from diabetes, for example) have decreased energy and are highly vulnerable to neurotoxic chemotherapy like the taxanes or platinum compounds. Many of the medicines used to control nausea (antiemetics) or decrease the side effects of certain chemotherapeutic agents are also potential neurotoxins. These include dexamethasone (psychosis and agitation), ranitidine (agitation), Benadryl, and some of the antiemetics (sedation).

Fatigue is a near universal complaint of older cancer patients. It is particularly a problem for those who are socially isolated or depend on others to help them with activities of daily living. It is not necessarily related to depression but can be. Depression is quite common in the elderly. In contrast to younger patients who often respond to a cancer diagnosis with anxiety, depression is the more common disorder in older cancer patients. With proper support and medical attention, many of these patients can safely receive anticancer treatment.

Heart problems increase with age, and it is no surprise that older cancers patients have an increased risk of cardiac complications (especially congestive heart failure) from anthracyclines and other potentially cardiotoxic anticancer agents. Because they are such effective drugs in treating the aggressive lymphomas, they are often used (safely, with careful monitoring) in all but the most high-risk group of cardiac patients. Patients treated with cisplatin chemotherapy require large amounts of intravenous fluid hydration. This can cause congestive heart failure in patients with heart problems; they need careful monitoring.

Lung (pulmonary) toxicity is sometimes caused by regimens containing bleomycin (like ABVD) that are used to treat HL. Lung disease is not uncommon in older people, and it is important to evaluate all patients with pulmonary function ("breathing") tests before starting bleomycin. A bleomycin-free chemotherapy regimen should be chosen for those with significant preexisting lung problems, and those at risk should have pulmonary function tests repeated at regular intervals during their course of therapy with bleomycin.

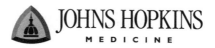

CHAPTER 11

TRUSTED RESOURCES—FINDING ADDITIONAL INFORMATION ABOUT LYMPHOMA AND ITS TREATMENT

Cancer Information Service of the National Cancer Institute
>http://www.cancer.gov/cancertopics/types
>/non-hodgkin
>(800) 4-CANCER

Listing of clinical trials as well as treatment options oriented for patients or health professionals. Try the health professional version for detailed references and evidence-based guidelines. You can request free information by calling their toll-free number.

The Lymphoma Research Foundation
>http://www.lymphoma.org
>(800) 500-9976

Links to informative sites.

The Leukemia and Lymphoma Society

http://www.leukemia-lymphoma.org
(800) 955-4572

Helpful fundraising tips. Free download of booklet called "Lymphoma: A Guide for Patients and Caregivers."

Lymphoma Information Network

http://www.lymphomainfo.net
(877) 897-5005

Patient-based forums and practical information.

American Cancer Society

http://www.cancer.org
(800) 227-2345

Clinical trials, treatment decision tools, and support programs and services.

American Society of Clinical Oncology (ASCO)

http://www.asco.org/
http://hematologicca.asco.org/
http://www.cancer.net/patient/All+About+Cancer
/Newly+Diagnosed/Find+an+Oncologist
(571) 483-1300

Find an oncologist and get up-to-date information on new developments.

American Society of Hematology (ASH)

http://www.hematology.org/
http://www.bloodthevitalconnection.org/find-a
-hematologist.aspx
(202) 776-0544

Find a hematologist.

Chronic Disease Fund

http://www.cdfund.org
(877) 968-7233

National Lymphedema Network

http://www.lymphnet.org
(510) 208-3200
(800) 541-3259

Free personalized websites

http://www.caringbridge.com
(651) 452-7940

Bringing family and friends together during a health crisis.

WHERE CAN I GET HELP WITH FINANCIAL OR LEGAL CONCERNS?

Accompanying any serious illness are questions and concerns related to expenses incurred as a result of treatment, health insurance questions that can be overwhelming to try to understand or resolve alone, and sometimes even legal questions related to employment or financial matters. Below is a list of national resources to aid you in addressing these types of concerns.

CancerCare, Inc.

http://www.cancercare.org
(212) 302-2400
(800) 813-HOPE
E-mail: info@cancercare.org

CancerCare is a national nonprofit organization that provides free, professional assistance to people with any type of cancer and to their families. This organization offers education, one-on-one counseling, financial assistance for nonmedical expenses, and referrals to community services.

National Coalition for Cancer Survivorship (NCCS)
> http://www.canceradvocacy.org
> (301) 650-8868
> (877) NCCS-YES
> E-mail: info@canceradvocacy.org

This network of independent groups and individuals provides information and resources about cancer support, advocacy, and quality of life issues as well as helps cancer patients deal with insurance or job discrimination and other related legal matters.

National Patient Advocate Foundation
> http://www.patientadvocate.org
> (757) 873-6668
> (800) 532-5274
> E-mail: patient@pinn.net

This organization provides educational information about managed care/insurance issues and legal counseling on debt intervention, job discrimination issues, and insurance denials of coverage.

The Leukemia and Lymphoma Society
> http://www.leukemia-lymphoma.org
> (800) 955-4572

Provides free information for leukemia patients and their families. Search for "financial support" on the website.

PatientAssistance.com
> http://www.patientassistance.com
> Not available by telephone

Non-profit information for the uninsured regarding programs and help.

Healthwell Foundation
http://www.healthwellfoundation.org
(800) 675-8416

Co-Pay Relief
http://www.copays.org
(866) 512-3861

Patient Access Network Foundation
http://www.patientaccessnetwork.org
(866) 316-7263

American Association for Retired People (AARP)
http://www.aarp.org
(888) 687-2277

Search by state for pharmacy assistance programs.

Needy Meds
http://www.needymeds.org
info@needymeds.com

Partnership for Prescription Assistance
http://www.pparx.org
(888) 477-2669

Together Rx Access Card
http://www.together-rxaccess.com
(800) 444-4106

Program for those not eligible for Medicare or Medical Assistance, with no drug coverage and limited income

Medicaid
www.cms.hhs.gov

Medical assistance for those with limited resources.

Social Security Disability

http://www.ssa.gov

(800) 772-1213

The Supplemental Security Income program is a possible resource for patients.

COBRA

http://www.dol.gov

(866) 487-2365

Information on continuation of health coverage after termination of employment.

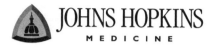

INFORMATION ABOUT
JOHNS HOPKINS

Patients with non-Hodgkin's and Hodgkin's lymphomas are managed by the faculty of the Division of Hematologic Malignancies at the Sidney Kimmel Comprehensive Cancer Center at Johns Hopkins Hospital. Visit http://www.hopkinskimmelcancercenter.org/ for more information.

You can also look up doctors by name or specialty here: http://doctors.hopkinsmedicine.org/

About Johns Hopkins Medicine

Johns Hopkins Medicine unites physicians and scientists of the Johns Hopkins University School of Medicine with the organizations, health professionals, and facilities of the Johns Hopkins Health System. Its mission is to improve the health of the community and the world by setting the standard of excellence in medical education, research, and clinical care. Diverse and inclusive, Johns Hopkins Medicine has provided international leadership in the education of physicians and medical scientists in biomedical research and in the application of medical knowledge to sustain health since The Johns Hopkins Hospital opened in 1889.

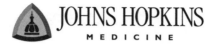

FURTHER READING

---

100 Questions & Answers About Lymphoma, Second Edition, Peter Holman, MD, Jodi Garrett, RN, Jones and Bartlett Publishers, 2011.

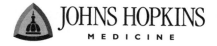

GLOSSARY

Adjuvant therapy: Treatment given after the primary surgery to increase the chances of a cure, and prevent the cancer from recurring.

Anaplastic large B-cell lymphoma: A type of aggressive lymphoma.

Anemia: Decrease in the number of red blood cells (can result in fatigue).

Anemia of chronic disease: Anemia caused by the bone marrow's reaction to being sick.

Ann Arbor Staging System: The system used to describe areas in the body affected by the lymphoma. It was created at a conference held in Ann Arbor, Michigan in 1972.

Antibodies: Specialized proteins of the immune system that help fight infections. They can also be created to recognize proteins on cancer cells; these are scientifically engineered antibodies that are identical (termed monoclonal) and are used in some types of lymphoma treatments.

Antibody therapy: The use of antibodies to treat cancer.

Antiemetics: Medications that decrease nausea.

Antigen: Any substance that can induce an immune response. This could be an infection or a cancer cell.

Anti-tumor antibiotics: A class of chemotherapy drugs.

Aorta: The main blood vessel (artery) that carries blood from the heart to the smaller arteries delivering blood to all parts of the body.

Aplasia: A condition where blood cells are not produced.

Apoptosis: A process by which normal cells die. Some cancer cells do not die, and a failure of cells to undergo apoptosis can contribute to the growth of cancer. It is often referred to as "programmed cell death."

Arteries: The vessels that carry blood containing oxygen to the organs and tissues of the body.

Autoimmune disease: An illness in which the person's own immune system can recognize parts of its own body as foreign.

B cells: A type of lymphocyte usually involved with immunity mediated by antibodies.

B symptoms: Fever over 38 degrees Centigrade (100.5 degrees Fahrenheit), soaking night sweats, and weight loss (greater than 10% baseline weight within 6 months) that may occur in lymphoma patients. They can occur individually or together.

Bacteria: One class of infectious agents.

BCNU pneumonitis: Inflammation of the lungs, and possibly lung damage, caused by the chemotherapy drug BCNU.

Bilateral: Both sides.

Biologic therapy: Treatment that utilizes immune system weapons on diseased cells.

Biopsy: A procedure in which cells are collected for microscopic examination.

Bone marrow: The soft substance inside many bones in the body where the blood cells are produced.

Bone scan: A nuclear scan that looks for signs of metastasis in bones.

Brachytherapy: A form of radiation therapy delivered directly by implantation of radioactive seeds.

Broviac catheter: A type of catheter that goes directly into a large vein to allow easier administration of medications and blood tests.

Burkitt's lymphoma: A very rapidly growing and aggressive type of lymphoma.

Cancer: The presence of malignant cells.

Carcinogen: Cancer-causing substance.

Carcinomas: Cancers that form in the surface cells of different tissues.

CD20: A protein on the surface of B lymphocytes and most B cell lymphomas. This is one of the favorite targets of monoclonal antibody treatment, such as Rituxan.

Cells: Basic elements of tissues; the appearance and composition of individual cells are unique to the tissue they compose.

Cellular immune response: The part of the immune response that uses lymphocytes (usually T lymphocytes) to directly remove antigens. In contrast, the humoral immune response uses antibodies to remove antigens.

Central nervous system: The brain and spinal cord.

Chemo brain: Difficulty with cognitive functioning as a side effect of receiving chemotherapy.

Chemotherapy: The use of chemical agents (drugs) to systemically treat cancer.

Chronic lymphocytic leukemia: The most common slow-growing type of leukemia.and also considered a low-grade lymphoma.

Clinical trial: A study of a drug or treatment in humans that appears promising but is not established as the standard therapy. Usually a clinical trial is done to improve the current standard therapy or procedure.

Comorbidity: A disease or disorder someone already has prior to a new diagnosis. Examples include diabetes, heart disease, and a previous history of blood clots.

Complementary therapy: Medicines used in conjunction with standard therapies.

Cyclophosphamide, doxorubicin, Oncovin (vincristine), prednisone (CHOP): The 4 drugs that are most commonly used together to treat aggressive lymphoma.

Cytogenetics: Laboratory examination of the genetic abnormalities in a cell. Cytogenetics is often used by the pathologist to determine the subtype of lymphoma because different lymphomas have different cytogenetic abnormalities.

Cytokines: Chemicals produced by T lymphocytes to generate an immune response.

Diffuse large B-cell lymphoma: A type of aggressive lymphoma.

Drain: A small tube inserted into a wound cavity to collect fluid

Epstein-Barr virus: The virus that causes infectious mono-nucleosis and can cause lymphocytes to grow abnormally. This virus may cause some cases of Hodgkin's lymphoma and several types of non-Hodgkin's lymphomas.

Field: The treatment site involved in radiation therapy.

Flow cytometry: A procedure for examining the proteins present on the surface of circulating cells in body fluids, usually blood or bone marrow fluid, to help identify the presence of cancer cells and the type of cancer. Flow cytometry is often used by the pathologist to determine the type of lymphoma in a specimen because different cancer cells have different abnormalities,

Follicles: Round structures containing lymphocytes normally located in lymph nodes.

Follicular Lymphoma International Prognostic Index: A modified form of the IPI (International Prognostic Index) for determining the prognosis of patients with follicular lymphomas.

Follicular lymphomas: An indolent low-grade lymphoma.

Follicular mixed small cleaved and large cell lymphoma: A follicular lymphoma with follicles containing both small and large lymphocytes.

Follicular small cleaved cell lymphoma: A follicular lymphoma with follicles containing only small cells with clefts in their nuclei.

Gallium scan: A nuclear medicine test that uses gallium to show areas of lymphoma within the body.

Graft versus host disease: An illness caused by the donor's immune system recognizing and attacking tissues and organs of the bone marrow transplant recipient.

Graft versus lymphoma: A situation in which the donor's immune system recognizes the recipient's lymphoma cells as foreign and works to eliminate the lymphoma.

Granules: Small particles containing enzymes.

Growth factors: Chemicals that can be injected to stimulate the production of blood cells.

Hashimoto's thyroiditis: A type of inflammation of the thyroid gland due to abnormal recognition of the thyroid gland as foreign.

Healthcare proxy: A document that permits a designated person to make decisions regarding your medical treatment when you are unable to do so.

Hematocrit: A measure of the number of red cells.

Hematologist/oncologist: A physician specializing in the treatment of blood disorders and cancer.

Hematology: The study of diseases of the blood, including blood cancers.

Hematopoietic stem cell: The most immature cell that develops into red cells, white blood cells, and platelets.

Hemoglobin: A protein present in red blood cells that carries oxygen.

Hickman catheter: An intravenous line that passes through the skin into a large vein near the heart. It provides a safer and easier way to administer chemotherapy and obtain blood samples.

Hodgkin's lymphoma (HL): A type of lymphoma, also known as Hodgkin's disease. HL can be classified into four further categories: nodular sclerosis Hodgkin's lymphoma (NSHL), mixed cellularity Hodgkin's lymphoma (MCHL), lymphocyte depleted Hodgkin's lymphoma (LDHL), and lymphocyte predominant Hodgkin's lymphoma (LPHL).

Immunoblastic lymphoma: An aggressive type of NHL.

Incidence: The number of times a disease occurs within a population of people.

International Prognostic Index (IPI): A system to determine the prognosis of patients with lymphoma.

Invasive cancer: Cancer that breaks through normal tissue barriers and invades surrounding areas.

Leukapheresis: A procedure that removes large numbers of white blood cells from the body.

Leukopenia: A low white blood cell count.

Living will: A legal document that outlines what care you want in the event that you become unable to communicate due to coma or heavy sedation.

Lymph: Fluid carried through the body by the lymphatic system, composed primarily of white blood cells and diluted plasma.

Lymph fluid: The fluid that carries lymphocytes around the body.

Lymph glands: The large collections of lymphocytes present at intervals throughout the lymph system. They can get big and painful in response to an infection. Also known as lymph nodes.

Lymph node architecture: The structure of lymph nodes when they are seen under a microscope.

Lymph nodes: Tissues in the lymphatic system that filter lymph fluid and help the immune system fight disease. *See also* lymph glands.

Lymphadenopathy: Enlarged lymph nodes, usually a sign of infection or lymphoma.

Lymphangiogram: An x-ray study of lymph glands after they are injected with a dye.

Lymphatic channels: The tiny vessels that connect the lymph glands.

Lymphatic system: A collection of vessels with the principle functions of transporting digested fat from the intestine to the bloodstream, removing and destroying toxins from tissues, and resisting the spread of disease throughout the body.

Lymphoblastic lymphoma: An aggressive, fast-growing type of lymphoma.

Lymphocytes: The main type of cell that makes up the immune system and is the abnormal cell in lymphoma.

Lymphokines: Chemicals that are produced by lymphocytes and help in coordinating the immune response.

Lymphoma: Cancer of the lymphocytes.

Lymphoma classification: A system to organize the many different types of lymphoma.

Lymphomatoid granulomatosis: A rare type of aggressive lymphoma.

Lymphoplasmacytic lymphoma: An indolent low-grade lymphoma associated with Waldenstrom's macroglobulinemia.

Malignant: A type of cancer that grows rapidly and out of control.

MALT lymphomas (Mucosa-Associated Lymphoid Tissue): A type of lymphoma that tends to involve lymph glands present in the mucosa (the lining of the gut or other organs).

Mesenteric lymph nodes: The lymph nodes present in the abdomen that anchor the bowel.

Metastasis, metastasize: The spread of cancer to other organ sites outside of its origin.

Monoclonal antibodies: A single clone of immune protein (antibodies) that binds to a specific target. Also known as monoclonal proteins.

Monocytes: A type of white blood cell involved with engulfing foreign proteins.

Monocytoid B-cell lymphoma: A type of indolent lymphoma.

Mortality: The statistical calculation of death rates due to a specific disease within a population.

Mucosa-associated lymphoid tissue: *See* MALT lymphoma.

Mutated: Altered.

Mycosis fungoides: A type of lymphoma that mainly involves the outer layer of the skin (the epidermis).

Neutropenia: A condition of an abnormally low number of a particular type of white blood cell called a neutrophil or a leukocyte. These cells play an important part in fighting off infection.

Noninvasive cancer: Cancer confined to its tissue point of origin and not found in surrounding tissue.

Nuclei/Nucleus: Structure within the cell body that contains the chromosomes and DNA of the cell.

Oncologist: A cancer expert who specializes in the treatment of cancer.

Palliative care: Comfort care provided to relieve the symptoms of cancer and with a focus on keeping the best quality of life for as long as possible.

Pathologist: A specialist trained to distinguish normal from abnormal cells.

Phases: A series of steps followed in clinical trials to ensure new drugs are developed safely.

Placebos: An inert treatment (such as sugar pills) given in clinical trials.

Plasmablastic lymphoma: A rare type of lymphoma due to immature plasma cells.

Plasma cells: The most mature type of B cell. They produce immunoglobulins and are the malignant cells in multiple myeloma.

Plasmapheresis: A treatment that consists of filtering plasma, the fluid portion of blood.

Platelets: Tiny blood cells that are produced in the bone marrow and are important for blood clotting.

Positron emission tomography (PET): Nuclear studies that use the abnormal sugar metabolism of cancer cells to identify metastatic deposits.

Post-transplant lymphoproliferative disorders: A type of lymphoma that occurs after an organ transplant, usually because the immune system is suppressed from medications.

Posttraumatic stress disorder: Emotional disorder resulting in a high level of anxiety and sometimes depression caused by a traumatic event in the past.

Primary care doctor: A physician who is designated as the principal manager of medical issues.

Prognosis: An estimation of the likely outcome of an illness based upon the patient's current status and the available treatments.

Protocol: The research plan for how long a drug is given and to whom it is given.

Radiation oncologist: A physician specializing in the treatment of disease using radiation therapy.

Radiologist: A physician who specializes in diagnostic studies to identify disease.

Red blood cells: Cells in the blood whose primary function is to carry oxygen to tissues.

Relapse: When cancer returns after a remission, requiring further treatment.

Retroperitoneal lymph nodes: Lymph nodes present in the abdomen that line the large blood vessels (aorta and inferior vena cava).

Risk factors: Any factors that contribute to an increased possibility of getting cancer.

Small lymphocytic lymphoma: A type of indolent lymphoma that is analogous to chronic lymphocytic leukemia.

Spinal cord compression: The encroachment of cancer cells into the spinal cord leading to compression of the spinal cord and the various nerves that go through it. Initial symptoms include the presence of sudden and progressive weakness in the arms or legs. This is a medical emergency and if it is not treated promptly could lead to permanenent paralysis.

Stage: A numerical determination of how far the cancer has progressed.

Superior vena cava syndrome: A condition in which the blood flow back to the heart is decreased due to obstruction, usually by very big lymph nodes.

Surgical oncologist: A specialist trained in surgical removal of cancerous tumors.

Systemic lupus erythematosus: A disease in which the immune system attacks the body.

Systemic therapy: A therapy or treatment usually given in the blood that affects the whole body (the patient's whole system). An example would be chemotherapy.

T cells: One of the major types of lymphocytes.

Targeted therapy: Treatment that targets specific molecules present in cancer cells, and does not affect normal cells or tissues.

Tumor: Mass or lump of extra tissue.

Waldenstrom's macroglobulinemia: A type of lymphoma that produces too much IgM (a type of antibody) and can be associated with an increased viscosity of the blood leading to symptoms such as blurred vision and headaches.

White blood cells: Blood cells that are most important for fighting infection.

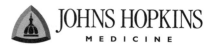

Index